T0235651

Watson's Caring
in the Digital World

Kathleen Sitzman, PhD, RN, CNE, ANEF, FAAN, is a professor of undergraduate nursing science, East Carolina University, Greenville, North Carolina. Previously, she was director of the Bachelor of Integrated Studies Program, Weber State University, Ogden, Utah, and a member of the faculty of the School of Nursing. Dr. Sitzman has been a nurse since 1983 and has produced scholarly work contributing to the body of knowledge of the nursing profession on the international, national, state, and community levels. She has been principal investigator or co-principal investigator on 10 research projects, several of which focused on nursing students' perceptions of caring online. She has received numerous awards for her scholarship, mentorship, and teaching, including the Jean Watson Award for outstanding scholarship in Caring Science from the International Association for Human Caring (2007–2008). Dr. Sitzman has published more than 100 peer-reviewed articles and has coauthored three textbooks: *Understanding the Work of Nurse Theorists: A Creative Beginning*, Second Edition (2011), *A History of American Nursing: Trends and Eras* (2010), and *Caring Science, Mindful Practice: Implementing Watson's Human Caring Theory* (2014, Springer Publishing Company).

Jean Watson, PhD, RN, AHN-BC, FAAN, is distinguished professor emerita and dean emerita, School of Nursing, University of Colorado, Denver, Colorado. She is the founder of the Center for Human Caring, Colorado; a fellow of the American Academy of Nursing; and a past president of the National League for Nursing. Dr. Watson is a widely published author and recipient of several awards and honors, including an international Kellogg Fellowship in Australia, a Fulbright Research Award in Sweden, and five honorary doctoral degrees, including Honorary International Doctor of Science awards from Goteborg University, Sweden, and from Luton University, London.

Dr. Watson's caring philosophy is used to guide new models of caring and healing practices in diverse settings worldwide. At the University of Colorado, Dr. Watson holds the title of Distinguished Professor of Nursing, the highest honor accorded its faculty for scholarly work.

Watson's Caring in the Digital World

A Guide for Caring When Interacting, Teaching, and Learning in Cyberspace

Kathleen Sitzman, PhD, RN, CNE, ANEF, FAAN

Jean Watson, PhD, RN, AHN-BC, FAAN

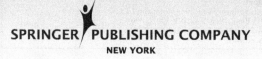

SPRINGER PUBLISHING COMPANY

NEW YORK

Watson Caring
Science Institute

Springer Publishing Company, LLC
11 West 42nd Street
New York, NY 10036
www.springerpub.com

Acquisitions Editor: Margaret Zuccarini
Senior Production Editor: Kris Parrish
Composition: S4Carlisle Publishing Services

ISBN: 978-0-8261-6115-4
e-book ISBN: 978-0-8261-6116-1
MOOC ISBN: 978-0-8261-6117-8

Ancillary MOOC teaching materials are available at springerpub.com/sitzman-mooc.

Printed by BnT

The author and the publisher of this Work have made every effort to use sources believed to be reliable to provide information that is accurate and compatible with the standards generally accepted at the time of publication. Because medical science is continually advancing, our knowledge base continues to expand. Therefore, as new information becomes available, changes in procedures become necessary. We recommend that the reader always consult current research and specific institutional policies before performing any clinical procedure. The author and publisher shall not be liable for any special, consequential, or exemplary damages resulting, in whole or in part, from the readers' use of, or reliance on, the information contained in this book. The publisher has no responsibility for the persistence or accuracy of URLs for external or third-party Internet websites referred to in this publication and does not guarantee that any content on such websites is, or will remain, accurate or appropriate.

Library of Congress Cataloging-in-Publication Data

Names: Sitzman, Kathleen, author. | Watson, Jean, 1940- author.
Title: Watson's caring in the digital world : a guide for caring when interacting, teaching, and learning in cyberspace / Kathleen Sitzman, PhD, RN, CNE, ANEF, FAAN, Jean Watson, PhD, RN, AHN-BC, FAAN.
Description: New York : Springer Publishing Company, [2017]
Identifiers: LCCN 2016034225 | ISBN 9780826161154
Subjects: LCSH: Nursing--Philosophy. | Caring. | Caregivers. | Internet in medicine.
Classification: LCC RT84.5 .S534 2017 | DDC 610.730285/4678--dc23
LC record available at https://lccn.loc.gov/2016034225

Printed in the United States of America.

Contents

PART **III**

Expanding and Continuing Digital World Caring

PART **IV**

Teaching Materials

Preface

Jean Watson's "Human Caring Theory" asserts that caring and love transcend distance, space, time, and physicality, and it is true. Feelings of love, kinship, friendship, grief, and compassion across time and distance confirm our basic shared experience of caring, regardless of physical and temporal boundaries. The rise of the Internet invites us to examine how deeply we believe in this transcendence, and challenges us to create new ways of caring in this increasingly digital world.

Understanding and explaining caring in the digital world—especially what it looks like, how to do it, and the day-to-day ordinary consistency of living it—is key to supporting an ongoing intention to care whether we can (or ever will) see, touch, or hear the beings with whom we interact. In this increasingly digital world, learning to care and love across distance, space, time, and physicality is critical to preserving the basic fabric of nursing and of humanity as we interact less *physically* but more *electronically*. We must all work together to envision and discover caring possibilities in the course of this inevitable change so that caring remains a core value in nursing and beyond.

The purpose of this book is to provide background and practices to support caring in the digital world. Educational activities and professional practice both rely on digital resources to facilitate interaction, collaboration, learning, and connection. Establishing a firm intent to care in digital settings and then enacting caring in ways that have been validated through research and other forms of knowledge development will help sustain caring as a core value in nursing and beyond.

This book has three major sections:

- Part I focuses on Watson's "Human Caring Theory" and how to generally apply the tenets of the theory in the digital world. The chapters in Part I offer an overview of Caring Science foundations, Caritas Processes, and examples of real-life applications and implementation strategies. *Readers are encouraged to read Part I first.*

- Part II focuses on specific approaches for teachers, learners, and professionals that have been shown to convey caring in the digital world. The chapters in Part II provide simple yet effective activities that teachers, learners, and professionals can do to support caring in digital learning environments and during everyday digital communications. These chapters can be utilized by readers in whatever order best suits their professional circumstances.

- Part III presents examples of initiatives aimed at establishing ongoing intent to care on the personal, local, national, and global levels. The chapters in Part III explore existing online free and open global educational opportunities related to conveying and sustaining caring in the digital world, and provide simple practices that will support personal and ongoing intent to care.

- Part IV consists of teaching materials for a self-contained course on caring that readers may use to create their own course on caring in professional or academic settings. These course materials also provide a concrete example of how to create clear and well-organized content for online courses.

- "Pearls of Wisdom," providing easy access to simple insights and activities readers may find especially helpful in understanding and enacting digital world caring, appear throughout the text. **Ancillary teaching materials are available at springerpub. com/sitzman-mooc.**

Kathleen Sitzman

Overview of Jean Watson's "Human Caring Theory" With Digital World Applications

1

Watson's Caring Science as Context for Digital World Caring

In this chapter, you will learn about

- *How Caring Science relates to the digital world*
- *Value assumptions of Caring Science*
- *Establishing a firm intent to care*

D emonstrating, communicating, and teaching caring are all expected components of nursing practice regardless of setting. "Caring" is "when the one caring connects with and embraces the spirit of the other through authentic, full attention in the here and now, and conveys a concern for the inner life and personal meaning of another" (Sitzman & Watson, 2014, p. 17). Within the nursing profession and other caring professions, "there lies a timeless ethic of caring and an honoring of the centrality of caring–healing relationships" (Watson, 1999, p. 21). This enduring caring ethic must be continually considered anew within the context of ongoing societal and technological change.

The rise of the Internet and the advent of continual, real-time, unfettered flow of thoughts, feelings, and information through electronic means have created an opportunity to envision and enact new ways of caring in the digital world. Watson foreshadowed this phenomenon in 1999:

> These [societal] changes fluctuate between intergalactic space explorations and digital world and hyperspace. They move between text and hypertext to hidden text, jumping from "word processing" to "thought processing," leaping from text to subtext to intertext; from actual to virtual, no longer aware of differences, no longer dealing with logical, linear thought or data. Such quantum leaps in human experience require that we reconsider our very concept of being. (p. xiv)

Watson's "Human Caring Theory" effectively accommodates these shifts in human experience by providing structure upon which an enduring intent to care can be crafted that will flourish and grow in the flow of ongoing change. Watson's Caring Science and 10 Caritas Processes help individuals, groups, and systems establish and nourish an intent to consistently care, and to engage in caring practices in any setting or discipline, whether face to face or in the digital world.

BASIC VALUE ASSUMPTIONS OF CARITAS PRACTICE

Watson's "Human Caring Theory" affirms certain value assumptions about the nature of caring. These assumptions form the philosophical foundation of Caring Science (Watson, 1985/1988, p. 32; Watson, 2008, pp. 41–42):

- If our humanity is to survive and if we are to evolve toward a more loving, caring, deeply human and humane, moral community and civilization, we must sustain love and caring in our life, our work, and our world.

- Nursing being a caring profession, its ability to sustain its caring ideals, ethics, and philosophy for professional practices will affect the human development of civilization and nursing's mission in society.

- As a beginning, we have to learn how to offer caring, love, forgiveness, compassion, and mercy to ourselves before we can offer authentic caring and love to others.

- We have to treat ourselves with lovingkindness and equanimity, gentleness, and dignity before we can accept, respect, and care for others within a professional caring–healing model.

- Nursing has always held a caring stance with respect to others and their health and illness concerns.

- Knowledgeable, informed, ethical caring is the essence of professional nursing values, commitments, and competent actions; it is the most central and unifying source to sustain its covenant to society and ensure its survival.

- Preservation and advancement of Caring Science values, knowledge, theories, philosophies, ethics, and clinical practices, within a context of Caritas cosmology, are ontological, epistemological, and clinical endeavors; these endeavors are the source of and foundation for sustaining and advancing the discipline and profession.

These assumptions are based on the following assertions:

- Caring and love are what power the universe.

- Caring is the central unifying force in the nursing profession, and in humanity.

- Caring is the primary reason for human existence.

- Self-care is critical in terms of facilitating one's ability to care for others.

Caritas Consciousness, Transpersonal Caring moments, and the 10 Caritas Processes described in Watson's "Human Caring Theory" are presented in Chapters 2 to 4 of this text. They provide a framework upon which individuals may build their own unique and sustainable caring presence/Caritas practice in face-to-face and digital world settings.

"Care and love are the most universal, the most tremendous and the most mysterious of cosmic forces: they comprise the primal universal psychic energy" (Watson, 1985/1988, pp. 32–33). This assertion is an invitation to build a personal Caritas practice that fosters constant awareness of the fundamental importance of caring and love in life and work. When making decisions in times of questioning or doubt, this approach acknowledges that love is ultimately the answer to every question. Consistently viewing Watson's work in light of this elemental understanding nurtures an intuitive feel for cultivating a personal caring comportment in self and others in any setting, whether it is face-to-face or in the digital world. Caring Science is concerned with human caring as it is expressed, explored, and experienced across a broad range of human occurrences. People are unified on infinite levels, with gross and subtle influences flowing in, around, and through all layers of existence. These influences emanate from individuals, to others, to community, to world, to planet Earth, to the universe, and beyond. Awareness of interconnectedness is a key component in caring interactions and activities.

Watson's "Human Caring Theory" is a philosophical and moral/ethical foundation for nursing that places a central focus on intentional caring at the disciplinary level. This model of caring includes art, science, humanities, spirituality, and continually evolving facets of mind-body-spirit medicine. Watson's "Human Caring Theory" is a guide meant to support day-to-day enactment of intellectual, physical, spiritual, and emotional caring for self and others through the establishment of a firm and consistent *intent* to care.

Pearls of Wisdom

Establishing and then consciously maintaining a firm intent to care is key to the process of manifesting a unique and enduring caring identity.

Watson's "Human Caring Theory" provides a theoretical foundation that supports discovery and knowledge in relation to dimensions of caring.

REFLECTIONS FROM JEAN WATSON: CARITAS CONSCIOUSNESS IN THE DIGITAL WORLD: CYBERCARING

In the 1980s, I heard Martha Rogers suggest that in the future, *Homo sapiens* would morph into *Homo spaciens*—recognizing that humans and technology are constantly comingling, evolving, and metamorphosing, transfiguring self and society.

At this point in human history, we are awakening to a reality that each person on planet Earth is part of a vast invisible veil and web with all of humanity and the environment. These advanced innovations are nonlinear, quantum jumps toward activation of social and human potentials—a universal humanity. Further, we are faced with a quantum leap in human consciousness, from physical to nonphysical, from matter to spirit.

Although we humans have learned, and continue to learn, how to evolve consciously with science and technology, we are challenged from within and without for survival of our basic humanity.

With these new human–technological challenges, we are called to apply values and practices of human caring and compassion to sustain our humanity and guide human consciousness evolution. Or we witness what Levinas noted: the totalizing and destruction of humanity (Levinas, 1969) and Mother Earth (Levinas, 1969).

As part of this evolution of technology and consciousness, we are entering a new worldview vital to ethical evolution and education, to guide us into the future.

Philosophies, ethics, and values of Human Caring Theory in education and practice can provide a guide for this new nonlocal consciousness and this new world, beyond the physical plane. Notions of transpersonal human caring (Watson, 1985/1988) can be used as a pedagogy–androgyny in the virtual world of education. Caring Consciousness radiating into the digital world has the potential to contribute to a moral community of human caring that honors, evolves, and expands the web of life.

Caring in the digital world—*CyberCaring*—unveils dynamics and relationships between transpersonal caring and advanced technologies, which point a way forward for global nursing education. By learning to combine a "one-world," "universal humanity" awakening with a shared global caring consciousness, we become part of quantum transformations contributing to the evolution of the human spirit and spirituality—thus, the evolved human.

REFERENCES

Levinas, E. (1969). *Totality and infinity: An essay on exteriority.* Pittsburgh, PA: Duquense University Press.

Sitzman, K., & Watson, J. (2014). *Caring science, mindful practice: Implementing Watson's human caring theory.* New York, NY: Springer Publishing.

Watson, J. (1985/1988). *Nursing: Human science and human care.* New York, NY: National League for Nursing.

Watson, J. (1999). *Postmodern nursing and beyond.* London, United Kingdom: Churchill Livingstone.

Watson, J. (2008). *Nursing: The philosophy and science of caring* (Rev. ed.). Boulder, CO: University Press of Colorado.

2

Caring Science Foundations

In this chapter, you will learn about

- *The meaning of mindfulness and mindfulness practice*
- *The nature of Caritas Consciousness*
- *The interrelated nature of Caritas Consciousness and Transpersonal Caring*

The term "caring" is so often associated with nursing and other caring professions that often caring is assumed rather than thoughtfully considered. Philosophical and behavioral dimensions of caring comportment must be examined, learned, and cultivated in order to facilitate the development of enduring reflexive skills. Caritas Consciousness and Transpersonal Caring describe two integral aspects of caring presence. Mindfulness practice in the tradition of Thich Nhat Hanh is one way to support the development of these critical aspects of caring.

MINDFULNESS AS A MEANS OF SUPPORTING CARITAS PRACTICE

Watson emphasizes that studying, reading, teaching, and researching dimensions of Caring Science is important work; however, to fully understand it, one has to personally experience it (Watson, 1999). Genuine caring calls for immediacy and full attention in the moment. Mindfulness practice in the tradition of Thich Nhat Hanh is not specific to any one faith or spiritual tradition, and can be helpful in supporting full attention and immediacy in Caritas practice. "Mindfulness is about letting go of doctrines and simply *being* fully present in each moment of life. *Ideas* about caring, understanding, and compassion are not understanding and compassion. Caring, understanding, and compassion must be *seen and touched* through the immediacy of mindfulness practice" (Nhat Hanh, 1993).

Mindfulness is consistently paying attention to what is happening in the present moment, moment by moment, and is helpful in cultivating deep caring and understanding. Staying aware of each moment sounds simple to do, yet it is challenging. Although our physical bodies are placed in the present, our minds and hearts often are occupied with the contemplation of thoughts, feelings, past events or future plans, and worries. In allowing our minds to be "preoccupied" in this way, we lose touch with what is happening around us in the *present moment.* Mindfulness is a practice that is meant to help unify mind, body, heart, and spirit with *what is happening right now* rather than what has been or what may be. In practicing mindfulness, we become fully available to see, understand, love, care, and enter the stream of what Watson describes as the "transpersonal caring moment." There is no time-defined path of caring, love, and mindfulness. Rather, caring/love/mindfulness is *the path* that manifests from the moment we fully attend to the present with the understanding that we are profoundly interconnected with all that precedes and surrounds us (Sitzman & Watson, 2014, pp. 25–26).

MINDFULNESS AND THE DIGITAL WORLD

How does mindfulness apply in the digital world? Mindfulness in the digital world is paying full attention to what each of us puts out and takes in from that world. We absorb and consume thoughts, speech, and actions that are conveyed digitally, and in turn, we produce digital materials that are consumed by others.

> The Internet is an item of consumption, full of nutrients that are both healing and toxic. It's so easy to ingest a lot in just a few minutes online. This doesn't mean that you shouldn't use the Internet, but you should be conscious of what you are reading and watching . . . . When you write an e-mail or a letter that is full of understanding and compassion, you are nourishing yourself during the time that you write that letter. Even if it's just a short note, everything you're writing down can nourish you and the person to whom you are writing. (Nhat Hanh, 2013, p. 4)

The energy of mindfulness supports understanding, kindness, wisdom, and sensitivity in the digital world. By mindfully

> letting go of judgement, returning to an awareness of the breath and the body, and bringing your full attention to what is in you and around you . . . [it is easier to] notice whether the thought [or digital message] you just produced is healthy or unhealthy, compassionate or unkind. (Nhat Hanh, 2013, pp. 4–5)

Mindfulness practice creates immediacy and spacious attention, providing the opportunity for caring to organically emerge from deepening awareness of *digital* interconnection.

MINDFULNESS PRACTICE AND TRAININGS

The following five trainings form a basis for mindfulness practice that will support caring (Nhat Hanh, 2006, pp. 14–15):

1. Reverence for Life

Aware of the suffering caused by the destruction of life, I am committed to cultivating the insight of interbeing and compassion and learning ways to protect the lives of people, animals, plants, and minerals. I am determined not to kill, not to let others kill, and not to support any act of killing in the world, in my thinking, or in my way of life. Seeing that harmful actions arise from anger, fear, greed, and intolerance, which in turn come from dualistic and discriminative thinking, I will cultivate openness, non-discrimination, and nonattachment to views in order to transform violence, fanaticism, and dogmatism in myself and in the world.

2. True Happiness

Aware of the suffering caused by exploitation, social injustice, stealing, and oppression, I am committed to practicing generosity in my thinking, speaking, and acting. I am determined not to steal and not to possess anything that should belong to others; and I will share my time, energy, and material resources with those who are in need. I will practice looking deeply to see that the happiness and suffering of others are not separate from my own happiness and suffering; that true happiness is not possible without understanding and compassion; and that running after wealth, fame, power, and sensual pleasures can bring much suffering and despair. I am aware that happiness depends on my mental attitude and not on external conditions, and that I can live happily in the present moment simply by remembering that I already have more than enough conditions to be happy. I am committed to practicing Right Livelihood so that I can help reduce the suffering of living beings on Earth and reverse the process of global warming.

3. True Love

Aware of the suffering caused by sexual misconduct, I am committed to cultivating responsibility and learning ways to protect the safety and integrity of individuals, couples, families, and society. Knowing that sexual desire is not love, and that sexual activity motivated by craving always harms myself as well as others, I am determined not to engage in sexual relations without true love and a deep, long-term commitment made known to my family and friends. I will do everything in my power to protect children from sexual abuse and to prevent couples and families from being broken by sexual misconduct. Seeing that body and mind are one, I am committed to learning appropriate ways to take care of my sexual energy and cultivating lovingkindness, compassion, joy, and inclusiveness—which are the four basic elements of true love—for my greater happiness and the greater happiness of others. Practicing true love, we know that we will continue beautifully into the future.

4. Loving Speech and Deep Listening

Aware of the suffering caused by unmindful speech and the inability to listen to others, I am committed to cultivating loving speech and compassionate listening in order to relieve suffering and to promote reconciliation and peace in myself and among other people, ethnic and religious groups, and nations. Knowing that words can create happiness or suffering, I am committed to speaking truthfully and using words that inspire confidence, joy, and hope. When anger is manifesting in me, I am determined not to speak. I will practice mindful breathing and walking in order to recognize and to look deeply into my anger. I know that the roots of anger can be found in my wrong perceptions and lack of understanding of the suffering in myself and in the other person. I will speak and listen in a way that can help myself and the other person to transform suffering and see the way out of difficult situations. I am determined not to spread news that I do not know to be certain and not to utter words that can cause division or discord. I will practice Right Diligence to nourish my capacity for understanding, love, joy, and inclusiveness, and gradually transform anger, violence, and fear that lie deep in my consciousness.

5. Nourishment and Healing

Aware of the suffering caused by unmindful consumption, I am committed to cultivating good health, both physical and mental, for myself, my family, and my society by practicing mindful eating, drinking, and consuming.

I will practice looking deeply into how I consume the Four Kinds of Nutriments, namely, edible foods, sense impressions, volition, and consciousness. I am determined not to gamble, or to use alcohol, drugs, or any other products that contain toxins, such as certain websites, electronic games, TV programs, films, magazines, books, and conversations. I will practice coming back to the present moment to be in touch with the refreshing, healing, and nourishing elements in and around me, not letting regrets and sorrow drag me back into the past nor letting anxieties, fear, or craving pull me out of the present moment. I am determined not to try to cover up loneliness, anxiety, or other suffering by losing myself in consumption. I will contemplate interbeing and consume in a way that preserves peace, joy, and well-being in my body and consciousness, and in the collective body and consciousness of my family, my society, and the Earth.

As the future unfolds, the need for steadfast caring in nursing and beyond has become increasingly apparent in the face of continual change and upheaval throughout humankind on local, national, and global levels. Caritas professionals will meet this need for caring at the individual, system, societal, national, and global levels.

Nurses with informed Caritas Consciousness could literally transform entire systems, contributing to worldwide changes through their own practices of Being, thus "seeing" and doing things differently—holding a different consciousness, radiating different messages, affecting the subtle energetic environment, spreading healing, wholeness, forgiveness, beauty, love, kindness, equanimity. In this awareness, nurses are literally becoming the Caritas field. (Watson, 2008, p. 59)

Pearls of Wisdom

Because mindfulness practice enables unbiased awareness of what is happening in the here and now, it supports accurate understanding and appropriate action in emerging situations throughout the day. Pausing and fully attending to one in-breath and one out-breath before reacting or responding provides an instant of full presence that will significantly enhance caring comportment and decision making.

CARITAS CONSCIOUSNESS

Caritas Consciousness and Transpersonal Caring form the underpinnings of each of the 10 Caritas Processes. Introductions to these aspects of Caring Science follow in the next two sections.

- Transpersonal caring moments, which will be further discussed in the next part, exist in the greater field of shared human consciousness.

- Transpersonal Caring moments are affected by the nurse's Caritas Consciousness—the studied awareness and committed stance in favor of caring.

- Caritas Consciousness affects the physical and nonphysical fields of existence for the caregiver, care receiver, and all others near and far in radiating circles of care and influence.

- The energetic field of Caritas Consciousness exists in, around, through, and beyond conventional understandings of time, space, and physicality.

- The person who cultivates Caritas Consciousness seeks immersion in a flow of awareness, thought, and interaction grounded in full attention, love, and altruistic intention toward self and others.

- The one caring is fully aware that the caring–healing process is dependent on interconnections among self, the one cared for, all other humans in the field of consciousness, and the higher energy of the universe (Watson, 1996).

- Recognizing that caring–healing–loving consciousness is not bound by time, space, or physical dimensions creates endless openings for envisioning and enacting caring and love in both face-to-face and digital world settings.

Caritas Consciousness is critical to teaching/learning, sharing, and interacting in the digital world because it ushers participants into a realm of human connection where seeking, acknowledging, and cultivating genuine caring is accepted, expected, and celebrated as a normal aspect of engagement in the digital world. Caritas Consciousness transforms the question of whether or not it is possible to care in digital settings into a quest for excellence in conveying and sustaining caring despite the absence of physical or temporal proximity.

Pearls of Wisdom

- *The development of Caritas Consciousness is enabled through the practice of mindfulness.*

- *Cultivate curiosity in all that you do. Unbiased, judgment-free observation in the moment facilitates the recognition of truth and fresh possibilities.*

TRANSPERSONAL CARING

Transpersonal Caring moments and relationships that emerge from the cultivation of Caritas Consciousness are the foundation of Caritas practice.

- Transpersonal Caring occurs when the one caring brings full attention and intentionality to the here and now and attends to the spirit and inner life world of the other. Together, the one caring and the one cared for build meaning and understanding based on authenticity, lovingkindness, and altruistic concern.

- Transpersonal Caring extends beyond the person-to-person encounter and influences the broader universal consciousness, enabling infinite caring connections and subtle interactive possibilities. These moments emanate ripples of love and caring into surrounding physical and virtual environments, like dropping a pebble into a pond.

- Opportunities to care that may have been otherwise overlooked become evident when one enters the stream of Transpersonal Caring.

  > The human care process between a nurse and another individual is a special, delicate gift to be cherished. The human care transactions provide a coming together and establishment of contact between persons; one's mind-body-soul engages with another's mind-body-soul in a lived moment. The shared moment of the present has the potential to transcend time and space and the physical, concrete world as we generally view it. (Watson, 1999, p. 47)

  The ability to holistically sense another person's state of being is influenced by whether or not the one caring has established a firm intent to care.

- With an established intent to care comes an awareness of the fleeting uniqueness of each moment, each situation, and each individual (including self).

- Every caring moment holds within it the kernels of wholeness and wellness needed in that very instance to facilitate the best outcomes possible.

- There is an old Zen saying that it is impossible to step into the same river twice, which illustrates the truth that each person/moment/situation is constantly moving, changing, and morphing from one form into the next in an endless stream of spirit, matter, and energy transmutation. This fluidity provides endless openings for genuine Transpersonal Caring moments to facilitate comfort, understanding, connection, healing, and learning moment to moment.

Transpersonal Caring moments are marked by full presence in the here and now with awareness of human interconnection that transcends matter, time, and space. Full presence as a sign of caring is not a new concept. Florence Nightingale became a revered public figure in England during the 19th century in part because of her strong and enduring commitment to paying attention to injured British soldiers. Here is part of a newspaper article written by John Macdonald for the *Times* (London) in 1855. It is about Florence Nightingale's work at a field hospital in Scutari during the Crimean War:

> She is a "ministering angel" without any exaggeration in these hospitals, and as her slender form glides quietly along each corridor, every poor fellow's face softens with gratitude at the sight of her. When all of the medical officers have retired for the night and sickness and darkness have settled down upon the miles of prostrate sick, she may be observed alone, with a little lamp in her hand, making her solitary rounds. (Bostridge, 2008, p. 252)

Macdonald's description of Nightingale's simple attention and lovingkindness is moving and inspiring. Readers in 1855 responded with great fervor and emotion, and deemed Nightingale a national hero.

- In the digital world, the ability to create and sustain caring moments is as critical as technological competency.

- Interacting, teaching, and learning can occur only within a series of nonproximal interactions, and caring connections are integral to the success of these endeavors.

- A caring moment in the digital world may be synchronous or asynchronous, with the utilization of text, voice only, or voice and video.

- Coming together by any digital means is an opportunity to create a significant interaction where connection can occur at the level of heart and spirit, thereby potentiating learning, and understanding of self and other.

Pearls of Wisdom

....we learn from one another how to be human by identifying ourselves with others, finding their dilemmas in ourselves. What we all learn from it is self-knowledge. The self we learn about... is every self. IT is universal—the human self. We learn to recognize ourselves in others ... (it) keeps alive our common humanity and avoids reducing self or other to the moral status of object. (Watson, 1985/1988, pp. 59–60)

Neither the broader universal consciousness nor the digital world is limited by time, space, or proximity. Conscious awareness of this parity opens a world of potential in terms of engaging in digital caring. Watson's Caritas Process no. 10, "Opening to spiritual, mystery, unknowns—allowing for miracles" (WatsonCaringScience.org, 2016), encourages openness and readiness to practice within this mysterious space of knowing and being. In the digital world, acknowledgment of the universal field of consciousness coupled with a firm intent to engage in Transpersonal Caring within this space allows for unbounded possibilities in terms of teaching, learning, interacting, and experiencing digital caring.

SUMMARY

- Transpersonal Caring occurs when full attention and firm intent to care are directed toward another human being whether the interaction takes place face to face or in the digital world, synchronously or asynchronously.

- Transpersonal Caring affects self, others, and the surrounding environment in widening ripples of influence that extend far beyond the initial situation, like dropping a pebble into a pond.

- Transpersonal Caring moments are the basis of conveying and sustaining caring in face-to-face and digital world settings.

REFLECTIONS FROM JEAN WATSON: FROM CYBERCARING CARITAS TO CYBERCOMMUNITAS

A *universal CyberCommunitas consciousness (digital caring community)* is now emerging from CyberCaring Caritas and Cyberlearning activities in the digital world. The following principles serve as foundations (adapted from Watson, 2008, p. 88):

- Each Caritas thought and each choice we make carries a spirit/energy into our lives and those of others

- Our Caritas Consciousness, our intentionality, our authentic loving presence make a difference for self and others, physically and nonphysically

- A loving mindfulness in our caring moments begets love and mindfulness for all

- Caring and love beget caring and love throughout the universal CyberCommunity, generating CyberCommunitas

- Caring and compassionate acts of love in the digital world beget healing for self and other, and lead to higher levels of consciousness for all of humanity

REFERENCES

Bostridge, M. (2008). *Florence Nightingale: The making of an icon.* New York, NY: Farrar, Straus, and Giroux.

Nhat Hanh, T. (1993). *Interbeing: Fourteen guidelines for engaged Buddhism.* Berkeley, CA. Parallax Press.

Nhat Hanh, T. (2006). *For a future to be possible.* Berkeley, CA. Parallax Press.

Nhat Hanh, T. (2013). *The art of communicating.* New York, NY: HarperCollins.

Sitzman, K, & Watson, J. (2014). *Caring science, mindful practice: Implementing Watson's human caring theory.* New York, NY: Springer Publishing.

Watson, J. (1985/1988). *Nursing: Human science and human care.* New York, NY: National League for Nursing.

Watson, J. (1996). Watson's theory of transpersonal caring. In P. H. Walker & B. Neuman (Eds.), *Blueprint for use of nursing models: Education, research, practice, & administration* (pp. 141–184). New York, NY: NLN Press.

Watson, J. (1999). *Postmodern nursing and beyond.* London, UK: Churchill Livingstone.

Watson, J. (2008). *Nursing: The philosophy and science of caring, revised edition.* Boulder, CO University Press of Colorado.

WatsonCaringScience.org. (2016). 10 Caritas Processes. Retrieved from www.watsoncaringscience.org/jean-bio/caring-science-theory/10-caritas-processes/

3

Caritas Processes 1 Through 5

In this chapter, you will learn about

- *Caritas Process 1: Embracing altruistic values and practicing lovingkindness with self and others*
- *Caritas Process 2: Being authentically present, instilling faith and hope, and honoring others*
- *Caritas Process 3: Being sensitive to self and others by nurturing individual beliefs and practices*
- *Caritas Process 4: Developing helping–trusting–caring relationships*
- *Caritas Process 5: Promoting and accepting positive and negative feelings yet authentically listening to another's story*
- *How each of the first five Caritas Processes can be expressed in the digital world*

aritas is a Latin word that means to cherish, appreciate, and give special or loving attention with charity, compassion, and generosity of spirit (Watson, 2008). The definition of Caritas is simple, but the practice of Caritas must be actively and consistently cultivated to be sustained and lived to the fullest potential.

Over the years, Watson has developed and refined 10 Caritas Processes™ to guide nurses and others in sustaining Caritas practice and cultivating caring moments/caring occasions in their own lives. The Caritas Processes may also be used to form philosophical and professional practice foundations at broader levels in clinical and academic settings. Caritas Processes 1 through 5 are presented in this chapter (WatsonCaringScience.org, 2016) along with digital world perspectives for each. Caritas Processes 6 through 10 are presented in Chapter 4.

CARITAS PROCESS 1: EMBRACE ALTRUISTIC VALUES, AND PRACTICE LOVINGKINDNESS WITH SELF AND OTHERS.

- Caritas Process 1 is about altruism and lovingkindness.

- The desire to altruistically help and care on multiple levels wherever possible is a hallmark of caring excellence in all areas of nursing practice, whether expressed in clinical, educational, or community settings.

- This altruistic approach begins with self and radiates to individuals, groups, communities, and beyond. Lovingkindness is an attitude and an intention that enables the adoption of an enduring intent to care.

- Varied behavioral expressions of lovingkindness emerge from this basic intent as individuals craft personal Caritas identities and offer their own strengths and gifts in support of caring consciousness.

- Each person embodies and demonstrates lovingkindness in his or her own unique way. There are many "right ways" to extend lovingkindness into the environment, depending on the situation, temperament of the one caring, and needs of those receiving care.

- Working from a foundation of firm intent to care that is tempered with mindful observation and consideration of key situational factors such as context, culture, and temperament will often clarify a beneficial approach to take.

CARITAS PROCESS 1 DIGITAL CARING PERSPECTIVE: TWO STUDIES RELATED TO KINDNESS IN HIGHER EDUCATION

- Clegg and Rowland (2010) pointed out that kindness in higher education is sometimes viewed as rather inappropriate "because the term suggests to some a 'sentimental and unrigorous approach' linked to 'leniency' and shallowness of thought" (p. 722). Clegg and Rowland also distinguished between "feeling kind" and "kindness" arguing that "considerable rigour is entailed in working out what would be kind in relation to the realization of the projects of others" (p. 724). In other words, lovingkindness can be manifested in a variety of ways depending on situational context. The most important aspect of enacting lovingkindness in this study was the *intent to be kind* in ways that were appropriate and meaningful for the individuals involved. This intent formed the underpinnings of approaches crafted to be suitable in terms of scope and tone for each situation.

- A study done by Cramp and Lamond (2016) identified actions that specifically communicated kindness in online learning environments (pp. 7–9):

  - Providing friendly and informal support and responses in digital social space
  - Structuring student goals to support student control
  - Designing online class sessions that ensure formative feedback can be used to improve assignments
  - Being dependably present online
  - Making recordings of course videoconferences to support student recall of critical information
  - Supporting students who are having difficulty transitioning into online learning

Cramp and Lamond (2016) concluded by saying:

> Our data suggest that being in digital spaces infused with the spirit of respect, trust, and responsibility (qualities we link to kindness because they help to see the experience from the learner's perspective) creates meaningful learning more successfully than approaches which do not prioritise [*sic*] kindness . . . We regard kindness as an essential element of the larger emotional landscape of [distance learning] and there are . . . strong narratives to support this view. (pp. 8–9)

Pearls of Wisdom

Research in online education shows that kindness, respect, trust, friendliness, and responsibility establishe a positive emotional landscape and support meaningful online learning experiences. Maintaining a firm intent to be kind is key in effectively enacting the first Caritas Process.

CARITAS PROCESS 2: BE AUTHENTICALLY PRESENT, INSTILL FAITH AND HOPE, AND HONOR OTHERS.

- Caritas Process 2 is about *paying attention.*

- When we genuinely pay attention to self and others, this simple act honors our shared humanity and instills faith and hope.

- People have a fundamental wish to be beheld, even if only for a brief instant. Can you remember a time when you felt unfettered attentiveness from another human being, when you felt truly *seen*? Those moments hold a special power to illuminate the reality that we are not alone and that deep interconnection is the basic fabric of humankind.

- Full and authentic presence is all any of us have to offer in any given moment because the past is over and the future has not arrived.

- In offering authentic presence, we are giving all that we have and all that we are to self, others, and the universal consciousness in that moment.

CARITAS PROCESS 2 DIGITAL CARING PERSPECTIVE: PAYING ATTENTION

There are many things in the digital world that vie for human attention, including:

- E-mail
- Texting
- Social media

- Gaming
- Internet searches
- Blogging

It is easy to move from one digital activity to the next without fully paying attention to any of it. Multitasking is also a common mode of functioning in the digital world. Inattention and multitasking are largely benign during solitary activities, but not so when others are involved. There is a difference between merely *responding* and genuinely *paying attention to* others in the digital world, and this difference is readily apparent to message receiver(s).

- How many times have you sent an e-mail message without the promised attachments, reviewed a sent e-mail only to find that you sent it to the wrong person, or discovered nonsensical words and phrases in a sent text message because you took the auto spell feature for granted and did not review the message before sending? These are all because of inattention.

- Oftentimes, inattention is apparent when we receive a digital message from a person who was not paying full attention when writing and sending it; perhaps there were simple misspellings; maybe the sentences were clipped or inaccurate; or perhaps the message referenced something that did not apply to you.

- Because we have become accustomed to interacting in the digital world, we are often able to readily pick up cues that hint at the level of attentiveness of the person who sent the message. Hiding inattention is more difficult than it might seem.

- Mindful cultivation of authentic presence for the few moments it takes to write and send digital communications is reflected in the quality of the messages you send.

- Consistently paying attention and offering full presence during moments when sending messages out into the digital world will instill faith, hope, and confidence in the receivers.

Pearls of Wisdom

Authentic presence described in Caritas Process 2 is predicated on the simple act of consciously paying attention. One of the highest honors you can give other persons is to pay attention to them.

CARITAS PROCESS 3: BE SENSITIVE TO SELF AND OTHERS BY NURTURING INDIVIDUAL BELIEFS AND PRACTICES.

- Caritas Process 3 emphasizes the importance of engaging in practices that support deep *spiritual knowing*.

- Centering, breathwork, yoga, prayer, immersion in nature, and other forms of acknowledging a divine mystery greater than ourselves are helpful in this endeavor.

- Specific spiritual traditions or nonspecific practices that hold individual meaning are integral to nurturing this aspect of self and other.

- In studying, practicing, and teaching Watson's theory over the years, I have found it helpful to incorporate mindfulness practice in the tradition of Thich Nhat Hanh into my daily flow of Caritas practice (Sitzman, 2002).

- Nhat Hanh's mindfulness practices are not religion-specific and can be cultivated within any spiritual tradition, or in the absence of spiritual tradition. "Mindfulness is the energy of being aware and awake to the present moment. It is the continuous practice of touching life deeply in every moment of daily life. To be mindful is to be truly alive, present and at one with those around you and with what you are doing" (Nhat Hanh, 2016). Authentic Presence, described in Caritas 2, mirrors Nhat Hanh's mindfulness.

Caritas Process 3 Digital Caring Perspective: Nurturing Individual Beliefs and Practices With Thich Nhat Hanh's Five Mindfulness Trainings

Adopting Thich Nhat Hanh's *Five Mindfulness Trainings* is one way to cultivate personal knowing/awareness that will facilitate growth and development in Caritas practice. Digital world applications of the *Five Mindfulness Trainings* are presented here (Nhat Hanh, 2009, pp. 35–38):

Mindfulness Training 1: Reverence for Life—Protect Life and Decrease Violence in Self, Family, and Society.

- Extend kindness and attentiveness to those with whom you interact in the digital world.

- Take measures to stop cyberbullying wherever possible.

- Support digital world efforts to spread peace and kindness to individuals, groups, communities, nations, and the world.

Mindfulness Training 2: True Happiness—Practice Social Justice, Generosity, and Nonexploitation of Others.

- Provide free and open opportunities for learning and fellowship in the digital world wherever possible, and support the efforts of others to do the same.

- Take measures to stop exploitation of self and others in the digital world by engaging only with organizations committed to fair and nonbiased education, socialization, and commerce.

Mindfulness Training 3: True Love—Facilitate Responsible Sexual Behavior to Protect Individuals, Couples, and Families.

- Support digital world organizations that promote sexual equality and responsibility.

- Take measures to decrease irresponsible sexual behavior through nonsupport of websites, blogs, and social media that promote it.

Mindfulness Training 4: Loving Speech and Deep Listening—Engage in Deep Listening and Loving Speech for Effective Communication and Reconciliation.

- Acknowledge the importance of attentiveness and loving speech in the digital world.

- Mindfully read and respond to cybercommunications with the firm intent to foster genuine caring, understanding, and reconciliation.

Mindfulness Training 5: Nourishment and Healing—Consume Only Those Things That Nourish Peace, Well-Being, Joy, Health, and Goodness in Mind, Body, and Spirit.

- Become fully aware of all that you are exposed to in the digital world.

- Carefully assess what you consume in the digital world and take measures to ingest only those items that engender peace, health, well-being, and goodness in mind, body, and spirit.

These five trainings encapsulate Watson's Caritas practices, especially in relation to altruism, lovingkindness, and the creation of loving–healing environments through mindful practice.

Pearls of Wisdom

Cultivating reverence for life and acknowledging the importance of love, happiness, deep listening, and mindful consumption in the tradition of mindfulness is one way to nurture individual beliefs and practices. Nurturing individual beliefs and practices facilitates sustained caring presence.

CARITAS PROCESS 4: DEVELOP HELPING–TRUSTING–CARING RELATIONSHIPS.

- Caritas Process 4 is about developing trusting relationships that create space and openings for Transpersonal Caring.

- A research project I did many years ago effectively illustrates how full attentiveness facilitates trust, Transpersonal Caring, and positive outcomes (Sitzman, 2001):

  - I studied an occupational health nurse at a large hospital who assessed office workstations to see if there was anything she could do to mitigate ergonomic issues that were causing repetitive stress conditions.
  - I had found from reading this nurse's satisfaction surveys that office workers who interacted with her were overwhelmingly positive about what she did to help them, and they faithfully followed her directives to permanently change their work habits.

- They expressed trust in her as a care provider, and this trust created resolve on the part of the workers to follow the interventions she suggested.
- When I asked these workers why they reacted so favorably to this nurse's efforts, I was astonished to find a powerfully consistent and simple answer: She paid close attention to each individual, pointedly excluding all other distractions during evaluation and intervention. These workers told me that they were certain this nurse cared because she *carefully listened and understood*, a hallmark of helping–trusting–caring relationships.
- She asked for input and repeated what she heard to ensure understanding. She mirrored facial expressions and physical actions, paying attention to each client fully and without distraction for the few minutes they spent together assessing the workstation.
- The interactions I documented required an average duration of 24 minutes, and in that short period, this nurse established *trust*, connection, understanding, and caring just by being fully present for those few minutes (Sitzman, 2001).
- This full presence, as described in Nhat Hanh's mindfulness, Watson's Transpersonal Caring, and Caritas Process 2, was instrumental in building the helping–trusting–caring relationships (Caritas Process 4) in the study just described.

Caritas Process 4 Digital Caring Perspective: Developing Helping–Trusting–Caring Relationships in the Digital World

I have learned from *being* an online student myself and talking with hundreds of online students over many years that trust must be earned in online classroom settings. Let me explain:

- When entering an online course for the first time, one is faced with a wall of technology and text.

- There is no earnest and trustworthy guide standing before you with ready answers and helpful demeanor to mitigate the anxiety of the unknown.

- If course materials are carefully and masterfully created, then trust builds. If the material is overwhelming, confusing, dull, or incomplete, then trust erodes.

- Trust builds and anxiety diminishes through the slow process of successfully navigating through layer upon layer of digital course material.

- If the instructor responds quickly and kindly to the reaching out of questioning students, then trust builds.

- If the instructor is sluggish to respond or responds with anything less than caring and concern, then trust erodes.

- If the student makes a poor effort to engage with the material, then the instructor's trust erodes. If the student makes an earnest effort to engage, then trust builds.

- If the student does not communicate with the instructor or does not respond to e-mails sent by the instructor, then trust erodes.

- If the student responds quickly with genuine respect and interest, then trust grows.

- If someone misses a step or accidentally steps on somebody else's toe, this will erode trust, but if it is swiftly acknowledged and corrected, then trust builds once again.

Such is the dance of trust in digital educational settings. The dance is never perfect, and everyone moves to the rhythms in their own unique ways. It can be helpful to remember that digital world trust is a dance with a few easy steps, and if the steps are followed, then trust-building becomes second nature.

Pearls of Wisdom

Steps to Building Trust in Digital Settings

- *Exhibit effort and excellence in crafting and posting/sending high-quality content.*

- *Communicate quickly, clearly, and often.*

- *When someone (self or other) makes a mistake, acknowledge and correct it with speed, forgiveness, kindness, and gentleness.*

- *Expect fluctuations in levels of trust, and have faith that genuine attention and lovingkindness will smooth them out.*

CARITAS PROCESS 5: PROMOTE AND ACCEPT POSITIVE AND NEGATIVE FEELINGS AS YOU AUTHENTICALLY LISTEN TO ANOTHER'S STORY

- Caritas Process 5 is about unbiased listening and creating spaces for self and others to express feelings without censure.

- Feelings need not be categorized as right or wrong.

- They emerge and pass away, disperse, and then re-form with speed and regularity, and none are permanent.

- Caritas Process 5 calls us to acknowledge, accept, and honor our feelings and the feelings of those around us.

- An infinite range of positive and negative feelings flow through the day-to-day existence of every person. With this realization come equanimity, gentleness, and forgiveness toward self and others.

- Feelings become less solid and frightening with the awareness that they will pass away as surely as they emerged, and that simply expressing feelings and then letting them move on is a healing act in and of itself.

- "The process of being with another in a nonjudgmental way as that individual expresses his or her feelings generates mutual trust and understanding" (Watson, 2008, p. 104).

- We are not our feelings, and those around us are not their feelings either. This awareness supports ease in letting go of impermanent feelings and helps facilitate recognition of and settling into the imperturbable ground of being that underlies every person's field of consciousness.

CARITAS PROCESS 5 DIGITAL CARING PERSPECTIVE: WAIT TO PRESS SEND

- Exploring feelings in the digital world is different than in face-to-face settings. The asynchronous nature of most digital world exchanges allows for careful consideration of what to say and how to say it if used to the best possible advantage.

- This means of communication can also pose challenges owing to lack of immediacy and inability to assess physical nuances when working through difficult issues.

- It is important to consider that positive and negative feelings expressed in the digital world create *digital footprints*, which are persistent artifacts that you have created as a result of your activities in the digital world.

- Anything you place on the Internet remains there indefinitely and can be potentially accessed and redistributed by others whether or not it was initially meant to be private. For these reasons, it is important to work with expressions of positive and negative feelings in the digital world with a great deal of mindful care.

Many years ago, when I first began teaching and interacting heavily on the Internet, I sent a few less than helpful messages and responses because of lack of experience and incomprehension of the effect my electronic communications might have on others. As I learned from my missteps, I created a few rules for myself and then made sure I followed them even in times of fatigue or frustration. My personal rules have cultivated self-reflection and helped to avert many instances where I might have produced less than helpful communications had I not paused and carefully considered my actions and responses in light of Caritas principles.

Here are my "Wait to Press Send" Rules:

1. When working with the expression of negative feelings, either yours or those of another person, make a draft of your message in a text document.

2. Leave the document for at least an hour, and then carefully reread it while referencing Watson's 10 Caritas Processes.

3. Ask yourself whether this draft demonstrates professionalism and Caritas practice.

4. Imagine yourself reading it out loud to a room full of professional colleagues. Are you comfortable or uneasy?

5. If your message reflects professionalism and Caritas practice, and if you feel good about the digital footprint it will leave, then send it.

6. If it does not, revise it, return to Step 2 and repeat the process.

Pearls of Wisdom

One significant advantage of digital environments is the opportunity to pause before reacting or responding. A brief but mindful pause encompassing one in-breath and one out-breath will support awareness of caring intent and help illuminate the best possible action to take in the moment.

REFLECTIONS FROM JEAN WATSON: CARING IN THE DIGITAL WORLD = CYBERCARING

Caritas Loving Consciousness in CyberCaring is universal; confined to no one spot, defined by no one way . . .

—influenced by Mary Baker Eddy (1821–1910), U.S. author, publisher, and founder of Christian Science

"CyberCaring" means caring in the digital world. It is a new concept; maybe we just made it up, like I made up the word "carative" as a counterpoint to "curative" in my first book (Watson, 1979/1985). So perhaps CyberCaring is the counterpoint to more mechanical meanings associated with medical technology, equipment, and commercial enterprises you may find on the Internet.

For example, if you Google "Cybercaring," you are asked:

"Did you mean: ***cybercalling cybercasing cyber calling cyberking***?" (Google: Cybercaring accessed January 30, 2016).

Thereafter, you find the word "CyberCare"—a multitude of organizations, largely for-profit, for biologically monitoring at a distance your chronobiology, your biorhythms, or physiological processes. Or there are home health CyberHealth for-profit telehealth companies to assist with monitoring equipment, electronic assistive technology. The other CyberCare identities are inspired nonprofit organizations in countries such as Philippines, Malaysia, and India, developed to serve underprivileged children or to fulfill a humanitarian cause.

The use of the term CyberCaring in education and online teaching as developed in this book has entirely different meanings and a more widely evolved, scientific–philosophical–ethical context as foundation: That is Caring Science.

As we enter into this unknown, yet known, Caring Science–CyberCaring world, a world designed to sustain and evolve Caritas loving consciousness for humanity, we enter a new world. This world of Caring Science–CyberCaring is unfolding, and being cocreated moment by moment with engagement by all the universal participants, transcending their engagement in chronological time and transcending their physical location on the planet.

Caring Science–CyberCaring is communicating/radiating caring/Caritas Consciousness beyond time and space and physicality—in harmony with the Universal Field of love. This is a world of one-universal-humanity.

REFERENCES

Clegg, S., & Rowland, S. (2010). Kindness in pedagogical practice and academic life. *British Journal of Sociology and Education, 31*(6), 719–735.

Cramp, A., & Lamond, C. (2016). Engagement and kindness in digitally mediated learning with teachers. *Teaching in Higher Education, 21*(1), 1–12.

Nhat Hanh, T. (2009). *Happiness.* Berkeley, CA: Parallax Press.

Nhat Hanh, T. (2016). Mindfulness practice. Retrieved from http:// plumvillage.org/mindfulness-practice/

Sitzman, K. (2001). Effective ergonomic teaching for positive client outcomes. *American Association of Occupational Health Nurses Journal, 49*(7), 329–335.

Sitzman, K. (2002). Interbeing and mindfulness: A bridge to understanding Jean Watson's "Theory of Human Caring." *Nursing Education Perspectives, 23*(3), 118–123.

Watson, J. (1979/1985). *Nursing: The philosophy and science of caring.* Niwot, CO: University Press of Colorado.

Watson, J. (2008). *Nursing: The philosophy and science of caring* (rev. ed.). Boulder, CO: University Press of Colorado.

WatsonCaringScience.org. (2016). 10 Caritas Processes. Retrieved from https://www.watsoncaringscience.org/about-us/caring-science-definitions-processes-theory/global-translations-10-caritas-processes/

4

Caritas Processes 6 Through 10

In this chapter, you will learn about

- *Caritas Processes 6 through 10*
- *Practical examples of how each of the second five Caritas Processes can be expressed in the digital world*

Caritas Processes 6 through 10 (WatsonCaringScience .org, 2016) in this chapter complete Watson's list of basic dimensions that support caring comportment in nursing and beyond. They are presented along with digital world perspectives for each. Although specific Caritas Processes may fit especially well into certain settings and circumstances at first glance, deeper study and consideration will reveal the applicability and importance of all 10 of the processes in each setting encountered.

CARITAS PROCESS 6: USE CREATIVE SCIENTIFIC PROBLEM-SOLVING METHODS FOR CARING DECISION MAKING

- Caritas Process 6 invites the use of full self and all available resources when working with challenging situations.

- Caritas problem solving emerges from curiosity and unbiased observation.

- All ways of knowing are needed to build understanding and create helpful interventions. These ways of knowing include empirical, personal, creative/aesthetic, and ethical/moral (Chinn & Kramer, 2011).

- True understanding requires the observer to mindfully employ multiple ways of knowing when planning caring interventions, interactions, solutions, and evaluations.

- Making caring decisions that will support the highest and most productive outcomes is possible when problem-solving methods employ multiple ways of knowing and are rooted in Caring Science.

CARITAS PROCESS 6 DIGITAL CARING PERSPECTIVE: CREATIVELY USING ALL WAYS OF KNOWING TO ASSESS INTERNET RESOURCES

- Problem solving that reflects Caritas practice must be based on reliable resources and knowledge development.

- The Internet provides readily available information that instructors, nurses, students, and clients use on a daily basis.

- Quick searches yield readily available tips and news. Professional or academic work is different. It requires in-depth, discriminatory searching in order to yield appropriately rigorous material.

The Internet has become a powerful, time-efficient, and indispensable source of constant information. The expediency of the Internet search process is so alluring that sometimes it is hard to remember that everything on the Internet is not necessarily accurate or true. This is especially important to consider in professional and academic work. Search strategies that employ all ways of knowing to discriminate between dependable and questionable sources of Internet information can be helpful in ensuring the quality of the information that you use. Here are some questions to ask when considering the use of Internet-acquired information:

1. *Empirical knowing:* Is it current? Does it contain references to reliable sources of information? What professional background(s) do the author(s) have? If it does not contain reliable sources and authors, and if the material is older than 5 years with no updates, then this may not be appropriate for professional or academic work.

2. *Personal knowing:* Does the information seem plausible and reasonable? Who is the intended audience? If it is other

than the one on which you are focusing your work, and if the claims on the website seem out of line with accepted knowledge in this area, then this may not be appropriate for professional or academic work.

3. *Creative knowing:* Is the information well presented in a professional manner? Does the site appear to be well maintained? Sites that are poorly presented or not regularly updated would probably not be appropriate to use for professional or academic work.

4. *Moral/ethical knowing:* What is the apparent intent of making this material available? Facts and information to help others learn? Sales? Persuasion to a specific way of thinking or behaving? If the source of information has the purpose of selling or persuading, then it may not be appropriate for professional or academic purposes.

Pearls of Wisdom

First impressions are not always accurate in relation to digital material. Check thoroughly before using. When assessing rigor and appropriateness of digital resources, be sure to employ all ways of knowing to effectively discriminate between dependable and questionable sources.

CARITAS PROCESS 7: SHARE TEACHING AND LEARNING THAT ADDRESS INDIVIDUAL NEEDS AND COMPREHENSION STYLES

- Caritas Process 7 highlights the importance of the teaching role in all areas of nursing.

- Nurses in clinical settings teach clients and one another on a daily basis.

- Nurses in academia teach soon-to-be nurses, one another, and clients in multiple settings.

- Caritas Process 7 encourages stepping into the frame of reference of the learner and *sharing* the teaching/learning experience, affirming that all involved have something to teach and something to learn.

- Genuine transpersonal teaching takes into account the whole person, the content, and the learner's readiness to learn.

- The meaning the content has (intellectual, symbolic, cultural, personal) for both learner and teacher affects the process of offering, receiving, processing, and retaining the content (Watson, 2008).

- Cultivating authentic presence will aid in identifying comprehension styles and personal needs of learners so that content can be conveyed in ways that support personal discovery, growth, relevance, and retention.

CARITAS PROCESS 7 DIGITAL CARING PERSPECTIVE: ADDRESSING INDIVIDUAL NEEDS FOR HUMAN CONNECTION

Interacting in the digital world is primarily text based because of the use of e-mails, phone texts, and asynchronous postings in blogs, wikis, and discussion boards. Caritas Process 7 calls us to take into account individual needs and styles, and then include strategies that will facilitate varied forms of interaction, sharing, and learning in the digital world. Alternate methods of communication and self-expression are readily available and should be used when working with learners who struggle with text-based interactions. Teachers, students, and professionals could do one or more of the following:

- Meet on the phone for one-on-one meetings.
- Use group conference calls for meetings with multiple people.
- Arrange and use telephone office hours.
- Encourage postings of images (photograph or artwork) or videos that demonstrate learning and new understandings.
- Meet using real-time video applications like Skype or Face Time.
- Use voice recordings instead of text in e-mail messages or postings.
- Provide access to digital educational videos for learning.
- Send out podcasts instead of newsletters to decrease dependence on written text.

As technology evolves, new methods of communication and self-expression in the digital world will emerge. Caritas practice requires willingness to continually learn about, use, and share new technologies that will aid in meeting individual needs and comprehension styles.

Pearls of Wisdom

Variety is key. Using a balanced combination of auditory, visual, and text-based communications will appeal to the individualized needs of the people with whom you interact in the digital world.

To enhance your understanding of the communication needs and styles of others, evaluate your own using one of the many available free online tools to assess communication or learning styles. Key phrases to type into an Internet search include:

- *Free Tool to Assess Communication Styles*
- *Free Tool to Assess Learning Styles*
- *Evaluate My Communication Style for Free*
- *Evaluate My Learning Style for Free*

CARITAS PROCESS 8: CREATE A HEALING ENVIRONMENT FOR THE PHYSICAL AND SPIRITUAL SELF THAT RESPECTS HUMAN DIGNITY

- Caritas Process 8 calls us to actively create holistic healing environments that honor basic human dignity.

- "Healing environments exist externally and internally, personally and collectively. Environments that promote healing and dignity tend to consist of elements that include [basic respect for all human beings], cleanliness, safety. . .collaboration, cooperation, beauty, kindness, orderliness, privacy, honesty, and holism" (Sitzman & Watson, 2014, p. 117).

- Mindful consideration of each thought, word, and action along with an understanding of the interconnectedness of all helps to diminish the natural tendency to feel above certain people/actions/situations.

- "Every act, every interpersonal interaction no matter how small or trivial, represents opportunities to promote dignified caring/ healing environments" (Sitzman & Watson, 2014, p. 117) in clinical, academic, community, occupational, and other settings.

CARITAS PROCESS 8 DIGITAL CARING PERSPECTIVE: CREATING HEALING SPACES

- Dignity and privacy, important aspects of Caritas Process 8, are also a critical aspect of caring in the digital world.

- Because it is so quick and easy to share images, posts, and texts in the digital world, privacy and dignity can be easily compromised.

- Guarding the privacy and dignity of clients by never discussing or posting images (full or partial) of them in any digital forum is an essential part of Caritas practice.

- It is also important to refrain from posting discussions or images related to colleagues, students, or faculty members.

Caritas Process 8 is also about creating healing spaces in the realms of mind, body, and spirit.

- When creating public/collective healing spaces in the digital world, Caritas nurses promote dignity through the use of respect, kindness, and honesty in interactions and content.

- Orderliness is facilitated through excellent design and organization.

- Healing and safety are supported through inclusion and staunch controls to stop bullying.

- Personal healing spaces in the digital world are best created by minimizing multiple or competing stimuli while cultivating mindfulness.

Here are some suggestions for how to use mindful breathing to minimize overwhelm and support personal healing spaces:

- Receiving phone calls or text alerts: Use the sound of the ringtone as a reminder to come back to the present moment. Breathe in with full awareness of your breath. Breathe out and respond to the message. Allow yourself to give full attention in that moment to whoever has contacted you.

- Texting: Breathe in, and determine the primary reason you want to send this text. Breathe out and create the message. Breathe in, and review the message to make sure it says what you intended. Breathe out and press "send."

- Placing a call: Before placing a call, breathe in with full awareness of your breath. Breathe out and resolve to give full attention to the person you are calling during the call. Breathe in and place the call. Breathe out with full presence and attentiveness.

- Interacting in the digital world: Breathe in with awareness that you are entering a social space. Breathe out, and consider what you want to contribute to this space. Breathe in with a firm intent to care. Breathe out and create your message. Breathe in, and review the message to make sure it says what you intended. Breathe out and post the message.

- Consuming digital content: Breathe in with awareness that you are entering a buffet of ideas, opinions, information, images, and constructs. Breathe out with resolve to place your precious attention on content that resonates with Caritas practice. Breathe in, and explore the digital landscape, returning often to the intent to care for self and others. Breathe out with gratitude for all that this digital world has to offer.

Pearls of Wisdom

Caritas Process 8 highlights the importance of facilitating dignity and wholeness in all environments, whether face-to-face or in the digital world. Pause and take one in-breath and one out-breath before acting. Cultivating this simple habit will support the clarity and perspective needed to create dignity and wholeness in virtual environments.

CARITAS PROCESS 9: ASSIST WITH BASIC PHYSICAL, EMOTIONAL, AND SPIRITUAL HUMAN NEEDS

- Caritas Process 9 is about seeing the sacred in the mundane, and recognizing that it is a privilege to assist others in meeting basic physical, emotional, and spiritual needs.

- Assisting others with basic needs yet cultivating an awareness of our own human needs, frailties, and vulnerabilities transforms the flow of ordinary everyday life into extraordinary Transpersonal Caring opportunities for healing, connection, learning, and spiritual growth.

- "Nurses help others manage predicaments related to the fact that human spirits reside in human bodies, and human bodies fail, wear out, and eventually die. The simple act of acknowledging this predicament [in self and other]. . .cultivates healing and wisdom in both the cared-for and care-giver" (Sitzman & Watson, 2014, p. 127).

- An important basic need for digital world users is the ability to safely and effectively navigate, communicate, and interact within this vast environment.

CARITAS PROCESS 9 DIGITAL WORLD PERSPECTIVE: ASSISTING WITH BASIC NEEDS OF THOSE WHO DO NOT OR CANNOT USE THE INTERNET

It has been documented that about 85% of American adults regularly use the Internet. The 15% who report *not* using the Internet do so for the following reasons (Zickuhr, 2013):

- 34% felt the Internet was not relevant to them.

- 32% were frustrated or found it too difficult to use, were physically unable to use it, or they were worried about virus/spam/hackers.

- 19% found computers to be too expensive to use.

- 7% did not live in a location where there was access to the Internet.

Because the Internet is a common fixture in society, it is easy to forget that up to 15% of the adults with whom we interact on a daily basis cannot or do not use it. Assuming that everyone with whom we come into contact uses the Internet, even though some people do not have the experience, knowledge, or resources to do so, could result in misunderstandings and miscommunications that will affect the fulfillment of basic social, emotional, and physical needs. For example:

- Many health care providers, social services, prescription services, and insurance providers require Internet connections to communicate, schedule appointments, share information, and process claims.

- Specifically asking health care clients whether they use the Internet will help clarify how best to meet basic needs in instances when Internet access is required to facilitate care.

- If a client does not use the Internet, then arranging assistance from a health care ombudsman or social services worker will ensure that the client has access to needed services through alternate means.

Likewise, many learners in online classes have limited or no experience learning in digital settings, which is a significant deficit in terms of basic needs and functioning in the digital world.

- Varying levels of assistance may be needed to enable inexperienced learners to complete course activities and requirements.

- Routinely asking learners to indicate levels of experience at the beginning of each course will allow for the creation of interventions aimed at supporting basic digital world functioning so that learning and academic productivity can occur.

Pearls of Wisdom

It is important to remember that the digital world is a distinct location of human activity and interaction where people have widely varying degrees of familiarity and comfort. Ask about levels of digital world experience and proficiency to clarify what measures are needed to support success in digital or online activities.

CARITAS PROCESS 10: OPEN TO MYSTERY, AND ALLOW MIRACLES TO ENTER

- Caritas Process 10 is about cultivating an open mind when it comes to phenomena that cannot be explained using conventional means of science or widely established human understanding.

- ". . . our rational minds and modern science do not have all the answers to life and death and all the human conditions we face; thus we have to be open to unknowns we cannot control, even allowing for what we may consider a 'miracle' to enter our life and work.

- This process also acknowledges that the subjective world of the inner-life experiences of self and other is ultimately a phenomenon, an ineffable mystery, affected by many, many factors that cannot be fully explained" (Watson, 2008, p. 191).

- Practicing this Caritas Process facilitates openings for unfettered exploration of the full human experience, yet acknowledging the mystery of life itself. It challenges Caritas nurses to cultivate awareness of this mystery and to allow self and others to communicate these mystical experiences without reservation (Sitzman & Watson, 2014).

CARITAS PROCESS 10 DIGITAL WORLD PERSPECTIVE: NEARNESS OF HEART

- The digital world offers many opportunities to cultivate nearness of heart with people who are far away.

- Texting, video calls, e-mail, and social media facilitate ongoing connections that would not have been possible before the advent of cell phones and the Internet.

- Caritas Process 10 invites us to appreciate and use digital opportunities to see and interact with loved ones, colleagues, and clients in an immediate way without limitations related to proximity.

- Cultivating nearness of heart through the sharing of text, sound, images, and videos is now a daily event in the personal and professional lives of many people.

- This opportunity to connect and reconnect with anyone anywhere through life's flow of constant change is one of the greatest miracles to emerge from the digital world.

Pearls of Wisdom

The mysteries of human connection, love, and understanding are fully accessible in digital world settings. If we are open to creativity and change, ongoing technological advances coupled with a firm intent to care will continually open new and exciting possibilities for caring across distance, time, and culture.

REFLECTIONS FROM JEAN WATSON: REMEMBER HOW WE MIGHT BE AFFECTING THE WHOLE

In the evolved consciousness of teaching and learning in Caring Science–CyberCaring, we have an ethical call, to pause and ponder our starting point. This awakening to our one world–one heart evokes moral arousal. We now know that our caring and loving consciousness and our purity of intentionality are starting points. Whatever we bring to the moment is affecting the whole and comes back to serve us or teach us.

Thus, teaching learning in Caring Science–CyberCaring moments, we acknowledge we are connecting with the Universal Field of consciousness – love energy – that connects with Infinity. The transpersonal CyberCaring "moment goes beyond itself, and becomes part of the history of each person, as well as part of the larger, deeper complex pattern of life" (Watson, 1985/1988, p. 59).

Again, it is well to remind ourselves that we never know in this consciousness how we may be touching the life of another person (Watson, 2008). The CyberCaring teaching moment can be an "eternal now" moment (Watson, 1985/1988, 1999) for another, connecting a lifeline of human caring to others, when most needed.

Finally, in this reminder space: Entering and engaging in Caring Science–CyberCaring in Education begins with the teacher being present, open to compassion, mercy, gentleness, lovingkindness and equanimity toward and with self, before one can engage and offer caring and compassion to others, locally or non-locally. CyberCaring teaching invites and evokes a contemplative, quieting down of the mind of the faculty and teaching moment with an opening heart to connect with One Heart, One World of Humanity. It is here through this grounding and moral arousal preparation that we can permeate the consciousness of our self and our world—contributing to the evolved human consciousness, radiating and manifesting a moral community of caring and kindness in the midst of a world in disarray.

REFERENCES

Chinn, P. L., & Kramer, M. K. (2011). *Integrated theory and knowledge development in nursing* (8th ed.). St. Louis, MO: Elsevier Mosby.

Sitzman, K., & Watson, J. (2014). *Caring science, mindful practice: Implementing Watson's human caring theory.* New York, NY: Springer Publishing.

Watsoncaringscience.org. (2016). 10 Caritas Processes. Retrieved from https://www.watsoncaringscience.org/about-us/caring-science-definitions-processes-theory/global-translations-10-caritas-processes/

Watson, J. (1985/1988). *Nursing: Human science and human care.* New York, NY: National League for Nursing.

Watson, J. (1999). *Postmodern nursing and beyond.* London, UK: Churchill Livingstone.

Watson, J. (2008). *Nursing: The philosophy and science of caring* (rev. ed.). Boulder, CO: University Press of Colorado.

Zickuhr, K. (2013). Who's not online and why. *The Pew Research Center.* Retrieved from www.pewinternet.org/2013/09/25/whos-not-online-and-why/

Conveying Caring When Engaged in Teaching, Learning, and Interacting in the Digital World

5

Conveying and Sustaining Caring in Digital Learning Environments

In this chapter, you will learn about

- *Applicability of Caring Science in digital world classrooms*
- *What nurse educators can do to convey and sustain caring online*
- *What learners can do to convey and sustain caring online*

Since 2001, I have been continuously involved in developing, revising, and teaching online nursing courses. During that time, I encountered many online educators who felt that it was impossible to convey, model, and sustain caring in digital classroom settings, but I disagreed. Caring and love transcend physical proximity, space, and time. Watson is firm in this belief (Watson, 2002), and I had seen it over and over again in my work with students, clients, and significant others, when genuine respect, love, and deep connection emerged or were sustained through interactions that took place at a distance. I was confident that this same transcendence would enable caring to be taught, modeled, and *truly felt* by teachers and learners in the digital world. Through direct experience, I knew there was great power in connecting with students at the heart level in digital classrooms, and I had observed and participated in the conditions under which caring and "uncaring" occurred in digital classroom settings. Digital instruction is a standard method of delivering nursing education, and it is critical that well-planned, intentional caring form the core of this endeavor. Research was needed to better understand the phenomenon of digital caring. Six research studies (Leners & Sitzman, 2006, 2010, 2015, 2016a, 2016b; Sitzman & Leners, 2006) confirmed that digital caring is possible and that certain practices tend to support it. In Part II, knowledge development from research done in online classrooms with resulting caring online guidelines will be presented in conjunction with corresponding Caritas Processes.

WHAT CAN NURSE EDUCATORS DO TO CONVEY CARING TO LEARNERS?

Establishing and then actively maintaining a firm intent to care is key to creating digital learning environments that convey and sustain caring. Intent to care sets the stage for creating structure and content that reflect Caritas practice.

General *attributes* of instructors who effectively convey and sustain caring in digital classrooms include (Sitzman, 2010, 2015, 2016a, 2016b):

- The skills necessary to write clear/well-organized communications
- An ability to sense when students need help
- A work ethic that supports promptness
- Mindful/empathic presence
- Ongoing engagement with students and course activities
- A high level of accessibility

An awareness of the students' frame of reference in relation to digital world learning is also important.

- The primary reasons students enter into digital world education overall are to facilitate career advancement or change, and to complete education/certification requirements for current careers (Aslanian & Clinefelter, 2012, p. 8).
- Students choose digital world over face-to-face delivery specifically because they need flexible course and assignment scheduling that can be balanced with work and family obligations and also because they want the ability to study anywhere/anytime (Aslanian & Clinefelter, 2012, p. 16).
- The majority of digital world students work part- or full-time jobs while in school. Respecting and supporting the basic needs of digital world students should be based on the knowledge that flexibility and family–work balance are foremost in the lives of these time-stressed working adults.
- Assignments and course activities should be carefully constructed in terms of clarity and organization so that students spend the bulk of their time meeting course learning objectives rather than figuring out how to navigate the course site or looking

for basic information that will clarify what the teacher would like them to do.

Specific *practices* in support of caring in digital world classrooms that have been identified in previous studies (Leners & Sitzman, 2006; Sitzman, 2010, 2015, 2016a, 2016b; Sitzman & Leners, 2006) fall into four areas, namely, *creating clear instructions, cultivating caring professional demeanor, sharing of self,* and *pursuing lifelong learning.* Discussion of these four areas follows.

CREATING CLEAR INSTRUCTIONS

The positive impact of posting clear and detailed written instructions has been validated in multiple studies (Sitzman & Leners, 2006; Sitzman, 2010, 2016a, 2016b) as one of the primary ways that digital world instructors convey caring to students. When an educator provides clear instructions, it allows students to effectively plan ahead, ask questions, and create a study routine. Clear instructions reflect kindness (Caritas Process 1), authentic presence (Caritas Process 2), trustworthiness (Caritas Process 4), respect for individual learning needs (Caritas 7), and consideration of students' basic needs to feel prepared and organized (Caritas Process 9). Specific activities related to creating clear instructions include the following:

- Course calendars detailing what students must do to successfully complete learning requirements

- Detailed rubrics that specify the length, format, and required components of all assignments

- Clear guidelines regarding acceptable social behavior (digital world etiquette)

Complete written course materials for an online class are provided in the Appendix. It provides concrete examples of how these practices might be demonstrated.

CULTIVATING CARING PROFESSIONAL DEMEANOR

Cultivation of a caring professional demeanor is an integral aspect of conveying and sustaining CyberCaring (Leners & Sitzman, 2006; Sitzman, 2010, 2015, 2016a, 2016b; Sitzman & Leners, 2006). Caring demeanor is expressed in the following ways:

- Responding to postings and individual communications within 24 hours during the work week

- Providing supportive/corrective guidance privately rather than in any public venue

- Conveying the belief that students will be successful in the online setting

- Recounting online challenges and solutions so students know they are not alone in their experiences

- Referring to specifics when commenting or responding so that students know their work and/or communications have been thoroughly read

- Providing scheduled phone availability

- Creating multiple contact opportunities to ensure availability when needed

- Giving weekly praise and encouragement to individuals and/ or groups for work that is well done

• Expressing enthusiasm for online teaching and learning

These commonplace activities are critical in demonstrating caring demeanor in the digital world. Responsiveness helps students feel valued and respected, cultivates trust, and establishes instructor presence and accessibility (Caritas Processes 1, 2, 4, 8, 9). Providing creative and sensitive guidance acknowledges the human vulnerability of students and demonstrates sensitivity to their challenges, needs, beliefs, and unique frames of reference (Caritas Processes 3 and 5–7). Enabling and enthusiastically engaging in multiple forms of digital world communication creates space for the miracles of significant connection, coaching, and mentoring to unfold among all participants engaged in the teaching/learning process.

SHARING OF SELF

Sharing of self supports CyberCaring (Leners & Sitzman, 2006; Sitzman, 2010, 2015, 2016a, 2016b; Sitzman & Leners, 2006) and is expressed in the following ways:

• The instructor will discuss past scholarly work and professional experiences where applicable in the course content.

• The instructor will post a personal introduction in the first week of class.

• The instructor will provide students with the opportunity for a face-to-face meeting at the beginning of the semester if possible. This can occur through videoconferencing if geographical distance prevents full physical presence.

Establishing human presence by making an effort to meet students face-to-face in whatever way is possible meets the real and basic need of many students to "see" their instructors in person at least once to cultivate familiarity and connection, and to satisfy human curiosity about how it feels to be in the physical presence of the instructor (Caritas Process 9). People feel cared for when they are truly seen, *beheld* by the other (Sitzman, 2001), and this simple activity establishes a baseline of connection and caring at the outset. Sharing professional and life experiences that add human depth and dimension, and encouraging students to do the same, creates openings for trust, kindness, understanding, and awareness of shared humanity (Caritas Processes 1, 2, 4, 7, and 8).

PURSUING LIFELONG LEARNING

Lifelong learning supports CyberCaring in online education by facilitating excellence in content creation and delivery. It is expressed in the following ways (Leners & Sitzman, 2006; Sitzman, 2010, 2015, 2016a, 2016b; Sitzman & Leners, 2006):

- Maintain proficiency in skills related to teaching within digital world environments by pursuing skill development opportunities and continuing education.

- Demonstrate ongoing expertise in content knowledge.

Instructors who maintain current expertise in technology are able to effectively use varied resources to mentor students through the online learning experience (Caritas Processes 7–9). Current content knowledge on the part of the instructor inspires respect and confidence on the part of the student, and provides a concrete example of professional caring at the disciplinary level (Caritas Processes 4 and 6). Overall pursuit of lifelong learning affirms a belief in the miracle of continual learning and renewal throughout the life span (Caritas Process 10). It also reflects commitment to excellence in professional roles, and projects a desire to provide the best possible education for students (Caritas Processes 2, 4, 6, 7, and 9).

Pearls of Wisdom

- *If a learner must fail an assignment, course, or program, then kindly enable the learner's dignity and hope by employing humility and creative problem solving to support a productive future.*

- Beginner's mind *describes the act of placing oneself in the shoes of another person. When creating course materials, employing* beginner's mind (i.e., walking in the shoes of students who have no idea what to expect or what to do) *will facilitate simplicity, clarity, and relevance.*

WHAT CAN LEARNERS DO TO DEMONSTRATE CARING IN RELATION TO INSTRUCTORS, PEERS, AND THE LEARNING PROCESS?

Digital world educators have identified specific student behaviors that demonstrate caring (Sitzman, 2015, 2016a, 2016b). Students can show they care about the course and the learning process by engaging in the following behaviors:

- Consistently demonstrating full presence through the creation of high-quality work and communications

- Communicating clearly, kindly, and respectfully with peers and instructors

- Reaching out to the instructor with struggles or concerns early rather than waiting until due dates have passed or tests have been taken

- Responding to instructor and peer messages within 24 hours

- Sharing personal and professional experiences that will enrich learning and understanding for all

- Pursuing learning with commitment and enthusiasm, which is evident by full engagement in the course with colleagues, instructors, and learning materials

- Acknowledging shared humanity of instructors and students

Clearly, kindly, and respectfully communicating with instructors and peers in a timely way inspires trust and demonstrates commitment and caring in relation to self, others, and the learning process (Caritas Processes 1–3). Verbalizing enthusiasm for learning and sharing experiences that will enrich the learning environment serve to foster appreciation for new knowledge and varied insights (Caritas Processes 2 and 4–7). Accepting the reality that self, instructors, peers, and colleagues are imperfect, and treating mistakes with gentleness and kindness helps to maintain a supportive space for self-discovery and the cultivation of deep knowing (Caritas Process 10).

Pearls of Wisdom

Examples of basic course materials for a 5-week training course in CyberCaring are provided in the Appendix. These materials are designed to reflect key practices related to Creating Clear Instructions, Cultivating Caring Professional Demeanor, Sharing of Self, and Pursuing Lifelong Learning. The materials include the following:

- *Instructor Course Plan Worksheet*

- *Syllabus*

(continued)

Pearls of Wisdom (continued)

- *Course Introduction*
- *Sample Instructor Introduction*
- *Course Calendar*
- *Assignment and Grading Description*
- *CyberCaring Etiquette Guidelines*

Please feel free to use them to teach your own course in digital caring, or as templates for creating/updating materials used in other courses to reflect caring practices.

REFLECTIONS FROM JEAN WATSON: CARING IN DIGITAL WORLD LEARNING ENVIRONMENTS

To take love seriously
and to bear and to learn it like a task,
this is what people need.
For one human being to love another,
that is perhaps the most difficult of all our tasks,
the ultimate, the last test and proof,
the work for which all other work
is but a preparation.

—Rainer Maria Rilke

This section has provided very theory-guided, yet very concrete, guidance for CyberCaring learning environment; how to develop and sustain Caritas Consciousness—*love*, both as teachers and students within a trusting community of caring and learning together—to deepen our shared humanity through a CyberCommunity.

One of the exciting aspects of even envisioning a CyberCaring community of learning is that you get to use your imagination; you get to imagine what others are thinking and energetically connect with them on their path. As Einstein noted: "Imagination is more important than knowledge."

As part of the one world/one heart awakening we each know we are not alone. In the CyberCaring learning environment, it is safe to imagine new ideas, creative possibilities, envision each other, united in a common bond and pursuit to personally know caring/Caritas/Transpersonal Caring more deeply—to actually experience it—trusting and knowing in your heart connection that you are touching others, and they you. You are not alone.

Remembering in your learning experiences, your thoughts and caring consciousness are transcending time and space and are connecting with the infinite field of Universal Love—the infinite field to which all belong. This reality is not just wishful thinking, but is now a universal truth of understanding the quantum universe. Everything in the universe is connected with everything else, out to infinity. This basic premise underpins Caring Science and the principles of Transpersonal Caring and healing.

Because of this reality of oneness—of a universal humanity—Cyberlearning honors this connectedness because we are all participants in one great web of life. Here we get to practice and personally experience CyberCaring and Cyberlearning.

Cyberlearning provides us with a sacred opportunity to grow in Love—to develop our intelligent heart. This learning opens us to a universal transpersonal Caritas Consciousness for self and others. As we engage in a Cyberlearning community trusting in heart learning, we affirm that the heart is the source of Love, caring, forgiveness, compassion, dedication, inspiration, creativity, hope, and trust. Our hearts are designed to express beauty, joy, our truth. As we more fully grasp Cyberlearning, we understand that perhaps at some level all our life lessons are in some respect learning more about love (Watson, 2008, p. 218.)

For example, if you are discouraged or depressed or feel frightened or confused as a student or teacher, you can ask for help from the universe and also, you can silently request guidance from your Cyberlearning community; you can review their postings; there you may find messages that are exactly what you need, messages that reinforce your hope and faith; there in Cyberlearning community, you are able to restore your confidence and your trust within yourself. Your peers and faculty may be your source of support and affirmation of confidence for following your heart.

Indeed, CyberCaring and Cyberlearning are new developments for humanity to evolve and grow to a higher level of consciousness—to come closer to living Caritas—Love for self and others.

David Hawkins, the renowned philosopher, scientist, and mystic, noted that the evolution of any one person toward a higher level of consciousness helps to elevate the consciousness of all of humanity; hence, this should be a reminder that whatever thoughts we put out into the field of infinity affect the whole. This is part of the shifting worldview from a mechanical and physical plane to quantum world thinking. This too is foundational to CyberCaring and Cyberlearning.

REFERENCES

Aslanian, C. B., & Clinefelter, D. L. (2012). *Online college students 2012: Comprehensive data on demands and preferences.* Louisville, KY: The Learning House.

Leners, D., & Sitzman, K. (2006). Graduate student perceptions: Feeling the passion of caring online. *Nursing Education Perspectives, 27*(6), 315–319.

Sitzman, K. (2001). Effective ergonomic teaching for positive client outcomes. *American Association of Occupational Health Nurses Journal, 49*(7), 329–335.

Sitzman, K. (2010). Student-preferred caring behaviors for online nursing education. *Nursing Education Perspectives, 31*(3), 171–178.

Sitzman, K. (2015). Sense, connect, facilitate: Nurse educator experiences of caring online through Watson's lens. *International Journal for Human Caring, 19*(3), 25–29.

Sitzman, K. (2016a). What student cues prompt online instructors to offer caring interventions? *Nursing Education Perspectives, 37*(2), 61–71.

Sitzman, K. (2016b). Mindful communication for caring online. *Advances in Nursing Science, 39*(1), 38–47.

Sitzman, K., & Leners, D. (2006). Student perceptions of caring in online baccalaureate education. *Nursing Education Perspectives, 27*(5), 254–259.

Watson, J. (2002). Metaphysics of virtual caring communities. *International Journal for Human Caring, 6*(1), 41–45.

Watson, J. (2008). *Nursing: The philosophy and science of caring* (rev. ed.). Boulder, CO: University Press of Colorado.

6

Expressing Caring in Digital Communications

In this chapter, you will learn about

- *How mindfulness enables caring communication*
- *Caring communication concepts and examples that will enable the creation of your own personal caring communication style*

D igital communications may either diminish or support caring. Context, tone, timing, and word choice all significantly contribute to the process of conveying and sustaining caring because moderating factors related to physical presence, such as gestures, facial expressions, and emotional presentation, are not readily apparent. This chapter presents communication approaches that have been shown to convey digital caring. These can be selectively used, adapted, and expanded to fit personal style and context.

CARING COMMUNICATION EXEMPLARS, MINDFUL COMMUNICATION, AND WATSON'S TRANSPERSONAL CARING

Research results validate the assertion that both caring and uncaring can be communicated in the digital world. A study completed in 2016 (Sitzman, 2016b) uncovered elements of caring online *communication* embedded within results from six previous studies aimed at identifying specific *activities* that elicited and supported caring in online classrooms (Leners & Sitzman, 2006; Sitzman, 2010, 2015, 2016a, 2016b; Sitzman & Leners, 2006). When caring communication elements from each of the six studies were analyzed together, a consistent pattern of digital world caring communication became apparent. Six distinct exemplars emerged (Sitzman, 2016b):

- *Offer full presence* by reading and responding to specifics in posts and messages, and attending to nuances in context, tone, word choice, timing, length, and frequency.

- *Acknowledge awareness of shared humanity* by discussing online challenges and triumphs, and by verbalizing awareness and understanding of shared human frailties and experiences.

- *Attend to the individual* by treating each person as a valuable human being with multiple dimensions that deserve love, attention, and respect.

- *Ask for and provide frequent clarification* by taking time to ensure that self and other(s) understand what is expected and needed from the other.

- *Demonstrate flexibility* through willingness to determine what will work best to achieve the most productive outcome rather than strictly adhering to rigid structure.

- *Point out favorable opportunities yet acknowledge challenges.* This can be expressed by sharing alternatives that will support moving forward with dignity yet attending to hindrances and difficulties with honesty and grace.

The study results also echoed key principles related to Watson's Caritas practice and mindfulness practice in the tradition of Thich Nhat Hanh, as described in Chapter 1. Table 6.1 shows parallels between the six Caring Communication Exemplars, Mindfulness, and Transpersonal Caring.

Pearls of Wisdom

The behaviors that support caring in digital settings are so simple and basic that it is easy to trivialize them and assume that they are a given if a person is generally considered to be "good," "decent," and "caring." The fact is that these behaviors must be consciously prioritized and consistently applied for them to be dependably demonstrated.

Table 6.1 Parallels Between the Six Caring Communication Exemplars, Mindfulness, and Caritas Intent

Caring Communication Exemplar (Sitzman 2016b)	Mindfulness Perspective (Nhat Hanh, 2013)	Watson's Transpersonal Caring (Sitzman & Watson, 2014)
Offer full presence	"I am here for you" (p. 73). I will give you my precious attention in the moment.	I will fully attend to you and your message through the use of authentic presence.
Acknowledge shared humanity	I am aware that you suffer, and I acknowledge that I suffer too. I want you to know that I am doing my best (adapted from p. 82).	I will create a healing environment for myself and those around me.
Attend to the individual	"I know you are there and I am very happy" (p. 75).	I will assist you with basic caring–learning needs. *You* are important to me.

(continued)

Ask for clarification	I want to understand and help (adapted from pp. 77–78).	I will cultivate lovingkindness for myself and others.
Propose flexible solutions	"You are partly right" (p. 83). We both have valuable perspectives and concerns to consider.	I will be flexible where possible through the use of creative problem solving and joint solution seeking.
Acknowledge challenges and point out favorable opportunities	"This is a happy moment" (p. 82). It is helpful to acknowledge challenges and to recognize conditions for happiness in each situation.	I will acknowledge and accept positive and negative feelings, and work to productively transform situations through caring. I will take time to listen to you.

Source: Adapted from Sitzman (2016b, p. 45).

PRACTICAL EXAMPLES OF CARING DIGITAL COMMUNICATION THAT OTHERS HAVE USED

Knowing the exemplars—the processes and attitudes that support digital caring—is helpful; however, finding the right words to use in everyday interactions can be challenging. In this part, the six Caring Communication Exemplars discussed in the previous section will be presented with corresponding phrases that others have used to convey caring in the digital world. These are starting points for creating individualized phrasing that resonates with unique personal style and context.

OFFER FULL PRESENCE

Offering full presence means paying complete attention to whatever is in front of you in the moment, and then moving on to the next thing and paying full attention to that too, in a continual flow of awareness. It is simply explained but not easy to do. Multitasking in the digital world is tempting because there is no immediate accountability in relation to focus or attentiveness. The quality and tone of what is conveyed will often reveal the degree of presence of the sender. These phrases, coupled with mindful intent to be in the moment, convey full presence (adapted from Sitzman, 2016b):

- I am here for you.
- My thoughts are with you.
- I am readily available during working hours via e-mail/text/phone, etc. and generally answer messages within 4 hours of receiving them.
- I am working online all day today—call/e-mail/text if you need me.

- I see you have sent a message that I cannot fully address at this time. I will respond fully by (day/time).

- I would like to talk with you. When can we connect?

- Sometimes it is helpful to see each other's faces. How about if we arrange a video call?

ACKNOWLEDGE SHARED HUMANITY

Acknowledging shared humanity involves a collaborative approach, where the recognition that we are all *human beings together* in this shared moment is the most important point to remember in every situation. Remembering shared humanity enables grace, forgiveness, kindness, love, and ease in self and others. The phrases presented here convey an understanding of shared humanity (adapted from Sitzman, 2016b):

- We are in this together.

- Let us learn from one another.

- I will do my best for you as we work through this together.

- Learning from mistakes is a normal part of growth.

- I have struggled with this topic, too.

- Timelines are challenging, but I also find them helpful to keep me on track.

- I can share with you what works for me if you are interested.

- If you will work hard to support your success, I will work hard to support your success, too.

- I know what it is like to get off track, and I think I can help you get moving in the right direction.

ATTEND TO THE INDIVIDUAL

Attending to the individual means letting the other know that his or her efforts, perceptions, and experiences are important and valuable. Individuals want to be seen, even if only for a few minutes (Sitzman, 2001). Individual attention, even in the briefest of instances, helps to instill motivation and sense of purpose. The phrases presented here convey individual attentiveness (adapted from Sitzman, 2016b):

- I want you to be successful.

- You are important to me.

- Your work is valuable to me.

- Your observations resonate with my own.

- I see you missed an assignment/deadline, which is not your typical behavior. . .

- You showed a lot of insight when you said. . .

- I missed seeing your contributions in the last discussion board/ online meeting.

- I really appreciate your attention to detail/promptness/sense of humor/sensitivity/experience/effort/diligence, etc.

- Please stay in touch. I enjoy working with you.

- I would like to know you better. Will you please tell me about your observations and concerns?

ASK FOR CLARIFICATION

Asking for and providing frequent clarification allows all involved to determine what is needed for success and productivity. An environment where clarity is openly sought and supported promotes growth, opportunity, and success for all despite differing talents, styles, and approaches. These phrases below convey a desire to promote clarity (adapted from Sitzman, 2016b):

- Do you understand?
- Do you need clarification or assistance?
- Is everything okay?
- Please talk to me about what you envision for this project/ assignment/situation.
- Are you prepared for the upcoming (meeting, test, assignment, presentation, etc.)?
- How is your day today?
- Is there anything I can do to help you right now?
- How are you feeling about. . .?

PROPOSE FLEXIBLE SOLUTIONS

Proposing flexible solutions is about attempting to understand the frame of reference of another person who may be struggling to understand what is expected or needed in a specific situation. It is also about assuming a flexible approach to problem solving when another person needs forgiveness or help. Flexibility in managing challenging situations engenders trust and hope for people who are struggling. The phrases presented here convey a willingness to entertain flexible strategies during a process of collaborative problem solving (adapted from Sitzman, 2016b):

- I am inviting input from everyone regarding how to make the project/assignment/rubric/test question(s)/instructions, etc. clearer. Please let me know your thoughts.

- I am having trouble understanding your written communications. I suggest we discuss things further in a phone call or video chat rather than by e-mail.

- Because you turned your assignment in early with good effort, I will give you an additional 3 days to redo the parts where content was missed.

- I would like to work with you to create a contract for completion so that we have clear instructions related to what you and I will need to do to move productively forward.

- Will you please share any ideas you might have about what might be helpful to get you up to speed? Maybe we can use them to create a plan that will work for both of us.

ACKNOWLEDGE CHALLENGES AND POINT OUT FAVORABLE OPPORTUNITIES

This exemplar is about acknowledging challenges in a straightforward way yet also sharing opportunities for growth and improvement. This approach supports moving forward with grace and dignity toward the most productive outcome possible. The phrases presented here acknowledge challenges yet also highlight opportunities (adapted from Sitzman, 2016b):

- I know you are struggling, but I would like to help and mentor wherever possible.

- Learning about this topic can be difficult. We have excellent tutoring/support/mentoring that will help.

- Although they can be challenging, group projects help cultivate collaborative skills that are critical to productivity in every working environment.

- I can sense your frustration/disappointment/sadness, and I am offering to work with you in order to better understand and help.

- We (or your group) productively worked together in this difficult situation and successfully found good ways to move forward.

Developing a caring communication style involves establishing a firm intent to care during every digital exchange, and then developing verbal and written habits that reflect the unique personality of the one conveying the words. It is helpful to assess context (circumstances and setting) when deciding what to say and how to say it. The example phrases presented in this chapter would be appropriate to use in a variety of settings involving the following:

- Caring communication between students and teachers
- Communication among colleagues in professional environments
- Communication between nurses and clients

Regardless of context, one simple well-placed word or phrase uttered with care and lovingkindness has the power to transform the phenomenal field face-to-face or in the digital world.

MINDFULNESS METHOD FOR CREATING CARING DIGITAL WORLD MESSAGES

Paying full attention in the moment while constructing digital world messages will facilitate caring communication in any context. The following steps involve just three complete breaths coupled with conscious intent to care. Doing this will enable the cultivation of full presence and centering, which are both needed to promote caring:

- Breathe in and carefully consider the purpose of your communication/content for both self and recipient(s).

- Breathe out and resolve to craft a message that will convey clarity and caring yet enable the highest and most productive purpose for this communication.

- Breathe in and craft your message with mindful awareness of the impact that even the briefest message will have on the people and environment involved.

- Breathe out and review what you have written, and envision who will receive your message. How will they perceive what you have written?

- Breathe in and add further clarity and caring intent to your message.

- Breathe out and send.

- If the message involves a challenging or delicate situation, refer to Chapter 3, Caritas 5 "Wait to Press Send" rules.

Pearls of Wisdom

The word choices presented in this section can be used as is, or they can be modified to resonate with personal style and professional context. Each example reflects movement toward what is wanted rather than what is not wanted. When communicating, it is helpful to use words and sentiments that summon caring impressions with a focus on going toward what you want (caring) rather than away from what you do not want (uncaring). This subtle shift in intention will guide the course of your exchanges toward caring.

REFLECTIONS FROM JEAN WATSON: CARING COMMUNICATIONS

This part provided concrete guides to philosophical–ethical and operational etiquettes and protocols regarding our consciousness, our communication, and our actions in the virtual Caritas Cyberworld. Electronic–digital communication evokes and invites a new awareness, an awakening, to the reality that whatever thoughts and responses we hold in our minds and consciousness, and even in our hearts, can affect the entire Universal Field—for better or for worse—for self as well as others. We can all benefit from guides to remind us to become more intentional, more conscious, and more mindful before we post or send electronic messages. It becomes a CyberCaring choice to pause and reconsider our informed moral actions in the digital world.

It is quite remarkable how a pause and thoughtful word and message offered with loving caring and kindness can literally, energetically change the phenomenal field for self and others. When we take time to offer a simple kind word as an authentic nonverbal gesture of concern and caring, we become a gift to the world.

The poet Anne Waldman reminded us "words are energy – they carry a physical and psychic . . . force" (Waldman, 2001, p. 178, in Watson 2005, p. 51). For example, emotions, thoughts, and words carry meanings at very different levels. Words and emotions we think of as negative, such as hatred, envy, anger, disdain, and fear, have a lower vibration—they are heavy and dense and lower the field; they separate us from each other and they hurt and close off the hearts of everyone exposed to them.

In contrast, words such as lovingkindness, concern, sensitivity to self and others, words that are encouraging and inspiring have the opposite effect: they speak to and open hearts; they unite; they lift up ourselves and others; we become lighter, eliminating some of the density of lower vibrations.

By the simple selection of kind and considerate wording of messages, we become a *living* theory and philosophy of CyberCaring in action, not just something to read about in a textbook.

The situation and the experiences are transformed through our simple, kind, thoughtful, and sensitive acts. As a result, we are sustaining and deepening our humanity, becoming more conscious, more intentional, more connected, more engaged, alive, open, authentic, and spontaneous.

Your chosen words of lovingkindness become sovereign expressions in your life, maturing your humanity and opening your heart with each kind message. Thus, you are simultaneously learning and practicing self-caring, self-healing; you are living out of the theory of Transpersonal Caring in a given cyber-moment. This guiding principle of cyber-communication opens you and us to the mystery of connecting and touching others in ways we can never know; and likewise, we allow for miracles in our life and work.

In summary, a CyberCaring methodology/pedagogy/androgyny practice seeks to sustain human dignity, basic civility, healing our humanity—which is caring and ultimately peace in action. We in CyberCaring are not just practicing Caritas; we become Caritas—living Caritas—humanizing hearts.

REFERENCES

Leners, D., & Sitzman, K. (2006). Graduate student perceptions: Feeling the passion of caring online. *Nursing Education Perspectives*, *27*(6), 315–319.

Sitzman, K. (2001). Effective ergonomic teaching for positive client outcomes. *American Association of Occupational Health Nurses Journal*, *49*(7), 329–335.

Sitzman, K. (2010). Student-preferred caring behaviors for online nursing education. *Nursing Education Perspectives*, *31*(3), 171–178.

Sitzman, K. (2015). Sense, connect, facilitate: Nurse educator experiences of caring online through Watson's lens. *International Journal for Human Caring, 19*(3), 25–29.

Sitzman, K. (2016a). What student cues prompt online instructors to offer caring interventions? *Nursing Education Perspectives, 37*(2), 61–71.

Sitzman, K. (2016b). Mindful communication for caring online. *Advances in Nursing Science, 39*(1), 38–47.

Sitzman, K., & Leners, D. (2006). Student perceptions of caring in online baccalaureate education. *Nursing Education Perspectives, 27*(5), 254–259.

Sitzman, K., & Watson, J. (2014). *Caring science, mindful practice: Implementing Watson's human caring theory.* New York, NY: Springer Publishing.

Waldman, A. (2001). *Vow to poetry.* Minneapolis, MA: Coffee House Press.

Watson, J. (2005). *Caring science as sacred science.* Philadelphia, PA: F.A. Davis Company.

Expanding and Continuing Digital World Caring

7

Expressing Global Intent to Care: Free and Massive Open Online Courses (MOOCs) and Trainings

In this chapter, you will learn about

- *Selected research studies that demonstrate personal, local, national, and global intent to care*
- *Free and open teaching–learning–sharing opportunities meant to foster dialogue, understanding, and collaboration related to caring*

K nowledge development in nursing and other disciplines indicates a movement toward intent to care on a global scale. Caring Science research provides evidence that Watson's "Human Caring Theory" is a catalyst for change in many settings—personal, local, national, and global. The studies highlighted in this chapter are from 10 different regions scattered across the world. They demonstrate the breadth, diversity, and global spread of settings where Caring Science forms at least a part of the underpinnings for research and transformative caring. These 10 studies represent only a fraction of past, current, and unfolding Caring Science research. Clearly, there is a transcultural/global movement toward informed and rigorous caring in health care and beyond worldwide. "In this emancipatory clearing for nursing and all health care practitioners, there is another movement towards the making of some common world: a world in which individuals and practice communities transcend traditional professional boundaries and come together to share unabashed love for caring and healing practices, integrating the human-nature-universe relationships in artful, aesthetic, healing practices and bringing together art, science and spirituality to a new depth for those engaged in healing work" (Watson, 1999, p. 19).

The Massive Open Online Course (MOOC) and caring on-line trainings that you will read about in this chapter are ongoing teaching–learning–sharing communities where anyone with access to the Internet has free and open opportunities to share experiences and perspectives related to caring. They provide forums for far-reaching awareness, dialogue, and cross-cultural/interprofessional collaboration related to deep caring in nursing and beyond.

EXAMPLES OF RESEARCH STUDIES THAT FOCUS ON WATSON'S CARING THEORY

- Childs, A. (2006). The complex gastrointestinal patient and Jean Watson's Theory of Caring in nutrition support. *Gastroenterology Nursing, 29*(4), 283–288.

This Canadian case study applies Watson's theory to the care of patients experiencing complex gastrointestinal disease. It was concluded that the application of Watson's "Human Caring Theory" facilitated holistic care that resulted in the best possible care for the patient.

- Clark, C. (2013). An integral-caring-science RN-BS nursing curriculum: Outcomes from fostering consciousness evolution. *International Journal for Human Caring, 17*(2), 67–76.

This article presented outcomes from an American RN–BSN program that implemented a curriculum based on integral-caring-holistic science to help students create caring moments and spaces for self and others. Educators in this program also grew in evolutionary consciousness as they taught this curriculum and collaborated with students in this healing–learning journey.

- Emoto, R., Tsutsui, M., & Kawana, R. (2015). A model to create a caring and healing environment for nurses in child and family nursing. *International Journal for Human Caring, 19*(1), 8–12.

In this article, participatory research was conducted in six clinical settings in East Japan to ask nurses to consider their working environments, appraise the caring–healing environment, and discuss concerns and new points of view. A process for facilitating the creation or improvement of caring–healing environments was created: interpret the present situation, expose hidden problems, express new points of view, share thoughts and experiences with coworkers, and perform care appraisal.

- Gustin, L. W., & Wagner, L. (2012). The butterfly effect of caring–clinical nursing teachers' understanding of compassion as a source of compassionate care. *Scandinavian Journal of Caring Sciences, 27*(1), 175–183.

This study, conducted in Finland, explored participant understanding of self-compassion. Findings revealed that self-compassion is a precursor to the offering of genuine compassion to others. Compassionate care involved becoming, belonging, and being together with another human being where mutual vulnerability and dignity were acknowledged, and compassion was a reciprocal event.

• Jones, M., Hendricks, J. M., & Cope, V. (2012). Toward an understanding of caring in the context of telenursing. *International Journal for Human Caring, 16*(1), 7–15.

This Australian study explored dimensions of caring in telenursing. Conclusions called for additional research because nurses' expressions of caring in telenursing are currently modeled after bedside caring practices rather than validated practices that are specific to the telenursing environment.

• Meng, M., Xiuwei, Z., & Anli, J. (2011). A theoretical framework of caring in the Chinese context: A grounded theory study. *Journal of Advanced Nursing, 67*(7), 1523–1536.

This study concluded that a caring framework based on Watson's Caring Science could be used in the development of integrative nursing curricula in China. It also concluded that the framework could be applied in evaluating clinical nursing and nursing education in China.

• Ogugu, E., Odero, T, Ong'any, A., & Wagoro, M. (2015). Nurses' and patients' perceptions on the importance of nurse-caring behaviors: A study at the surgical wards of Kenyatta National Hospital, Nairobi. *International Journal for Human Caring, 19*(2), 55–61.

This study, conducted at a hospital in Nairobi, compared nurse and patient perceptions on the importance of nurse-caring behaviors. The theoretical framework for the study was Watson's

"Human Caring Theory." Results showed differing perceptions of what caring behaviors were most important. Nurses valued treating the patients as individuals and having the ability to administer injections as most important. Patients valued on-time treatments and medication administration, and assisting with care until reaching independence to be the most valuable caring behaviors. It was suggested that patient care protocols within the hospital be adjusted to prioritize patient preferences.

- Ozkan, I. A., Okumus, H., Buldukoglu, K., & Watson, J. (2013). A case study based on Watson's Theory of Human Caring: Being an infertile woman in Turkey. *Nursing Science Quarterly, 26*(4), 352–359.

   This article details a case study completed in Turkey with infertile women and the nurses who work with them. It was determined that applying Watson's theory was useful and relevant in planning and engaging in care for this population in terms of maintaining a therapeutic environment.

- Santos, M. R., Bousso, R. S., Vendramim, P., Baliza, M. F., Misko, M. D., & Silva, L. (2014). The practice of nurses caring for families of pediatric inpatients in light of Jean Watson. *Revista da Escola de Enfermagem da USP, 48*(Esp), 80–86.

   This Brazilian study found that Watson's Caring Science could be used in an inpatient pediatric setting to aid in establishing a caring culture. Nurses in the study recognized the usefulness of incorporating Caring Science practice elements into their work with patients and families in order to improve interpersonal and caring relations.

- Suliman, W. A., Welmann, E., Omer, T., & Thomas, L. (2009). Applying Watson's Nursing Theory to assess patient perceptions of being cared for in a multicultural environment. *Journal of Nursing Research, 17*(4), 293–300.

This study, done in the Middle East, concluded that caring behaviors based on Watson's Caring Science were valued by Saudi patients regardless of cultural differences with their caregivers. Recommendations were made to base nursing care on principles of Caring Science in order to meet patient needs.

WHAT IS A MASSIVE OPEN ONLINE COURSE (MOOC), AND HOW MIGHT ONE BE USED TO SUPPORT GLOBAL DIGITAL CARING?

MOOCs are noncredit courses offered free by universities or organizations to anyone interested in enrolling.

- The only requirement is that registrants must have access to the Internet. People who register need not have any formal affiliation with the university or organization offering the MOOC.

- MOOCs started appearing around 2008, and MOOC offerings increased dramatically in 2011 when professors from Stanford University (U.S.) released MOOC educational videos and free web resources, and then later established an independent for-profit technology called "Coursera" to support the creation of MOOCs (Baturay, 2015).

- The number of MOOCs worldwide surged in 2011 and 2012, but later began to decrease as the MOOC concept and technology matured and settled into the broader educational landscape.

- Today, MOOCs are offered on multiple platforms around the world and address a wide range of subject areas.

- They continue to provide large open forums for participants to learn about topics of common interest in structured and collaborative learning environments.

- Dialogue about how MOOCs can best be used to provide educational opportunities at the local, national, and global levels, yet still preserving traditional educational practices, is ongoing (Brahimi & Sarirete, 2014).

Because the Caring Science community of students, educators, scholars, and professionals incudes people with Internet access all over the world, I began to consider the possibility that a Caring Science MOOC could be one way to reach out and provide collective opportunities for connection, inspiration, and continuity—CyberCommunitas—which is an integral component of establishing global caring consciousness because

- MOOCs and other free and open digital world endeavors provide opportunities for ongoing connections and exchange of ideas among those who are interested in furthering deep caring in self, others, communities, nations, and the world;

- Free and open digital world gatherings transcend geography, economic limitations, and sociopolitical conditions that would otherwise hinder the development of significant connections, interactions, and collaborations.

In an effort to create a caring–learning–collaborative space for people to learn about Caring Science, and to openly explore feelings, observations, questions, and experiences in caring, I formed a collaboration that included East Carolina University (North Carolina), Weber State University (Utah), University of Colorado-Denver (Colorado), Watson Caring Science Institute (Colorado), and Canvas/Instructure Learning Management System (Utah), and created a MOOC entitled "Caring Science, Mindful Practice: Implementing Watson's 'Human Caring Theory,' " offered free of charge twice a year to anyone, worldwide, with access to the Internet (canvas.net).

- The purpose of the course is to provide tools to facilitate professional caring practices in everyday work environments.
- Learners are introduced to Watson's "Human Caring Theory" and then asked to communicate their own experiences related to caring throughout the course.
- Exploration and learning related to key concepts are supported through the introduction of mindfulness practice, reflective narrative, and contemplative art.
- Asynchronous discussion, moderated by a team of educators knowledgeable in Caring Science, provides a forum for on-going interaction and discovery among participants during each 4-week class session.
- Certificates of completion are earned by participants who complete all the course learning modules.

On completion of the course, the students should be able to do the following:

- Explain Watson's 10 Caritas Processes.
- Describe how mindfulness practice might be useful in supporting deepened understanding and practice of Caring Science.
- Provide professional examples that illustrate Watson's 10 Caritas Processes.
- Provide professional examples that illustrate Transpersonal Caring moments.
- Discuss how Watson's Caritas Consciousness touchstones for cultivating love might be useful in everyday professional caring practice.

Teaching Strategies include the following:

- Course-specific reading materials in print and/or online formats
- Asynchronous online postings and discussion boards
- Online reflective journaling
- Multimedia presentations as appropriate in the online setting

    Topical areas include the following:

- Mindfulness and cultivating understanding of Watson's "Human Caring Theory"
- Overview of Watson's Theory
- Thich Nhat Hanh's *Five Mindfulness Trainings*
- Transpersonal Caring moments
- The 10 Caritas Processes
- Caritas Consciousness touchstones for cultivating love

The class is pass/fail. Students earning 80% of the total points available in the course receive a passing grade and earn the corresponding certificate of completion.

In addition to web links, video lectures, slide presentations, and instructional materials, there is a textbook available to accompany the course:

- Sitzman, K., & Watson, J. (2014). *Caring Science, Mindful Practice*. New York, NY: Springer Publishing.

To date, more than 1,700 people from all over the world have registered for the course. Learners have come from:

- The United States
- Western Europe

- The South Pacific
- Africa
- South Asia
- The Middle East
- Southeast Asia
- East Asia

Other demographic information has shown the following:

- The majority of the participants so far have spoken English; however, non-English speakers have used Google Translate or other free Internet-based translation service to participate effectively within the required discussion boards.
- Students' educational backgrounds have ranged from doctoral degrees to high school diplomas and everything in between.
- Although, in terms of occupational background, nurses and allied health professionals made up the bulk of the students, many outside of nursing have also joined. They came from professions as diverse as engineering, retail sales, elementary education, advertising, executive assisting, and many others.

Multiple volunteer Caritas faculty members within this MOOC ensured that students had continual support and guidance as they worked through 4 weeks of Caring Science content. Outcomes related to the MOOC have been highly favorable:

- Student work was insightful and demonstrated commitment to learning and real-world application of Caring Science.

- The asynchronous discussion board posting areas were supportive, creative, and inclusive spaces where experiences, observations, and insights were shared among faculty and participants.

- Enduring connections that crossed cultures, languages, and geographical distances were formed among participants. Students continually expressed gratitude for the opportunity to communicate with others about deep caring without censure in an open and nurturing environment.

- Data from student course evaluations completed after the first offering were overwhelmingly positive, with 95% of the respondents giving the course a rating of five stars (70%) or 4 stars (25%) out of a possible five stars for overall satisfaction with the learning/collaborative experience.

This course will be offered into the future as an ongoing space for Caring Science learning, sharing, and collaborating.

Pearls of Wisdom

The success of the Caring Science, Mindful Practice MOOC has demonstrated that there is a global need for open access content related to caring and caring professions. We also learned that it is possible to effectively overcome language and cultural challenges in global classrooms through the use of currently available free technology. Learners uniformly expressed appreciation for opportunities to interact with and learn from others in globally diverse classroom settings, and also expressed a desire to carry new knowledge and understanding about Caring Science into work and life.

FREE AND OPEN TRAININGS TO SUPPORT DIGITAL CARING LOCALLY AND GLOBALLY

The free and open online training opportunities discussed here are self-guided and asynchronous, so that anyone with access to the Internet can benefit from free learning/training opportunities that are self-paced. In this way, the tremendous value of lifelong learning can be offered to a wide audience. The trainings are situated within the Office of Faculty Excellence at East Carolina University (ECU), where outreach and community service are deeply valued. The trainings are available to people who are affiliated with ECU, and also to anyone outside the university who is interested in learning about how to convey and sustain caring in digital settings. The titles of the trainings are:

- Conveying and Sustaining Caring in Online Classrooms
- Mindful Communication for Caring Online

   The content of both trainings is based on the six previously discussed research studies related to conveying and sustaining caring online.

- Direct links to both trainings are provided on the publicly visible ECU Office of Faculty Excellence website.
- The trainings are structured as interactive narrated slide presentations.
- Each training requires 45 minutes to an hour to complete for most people, although learners are permitted to take as much time as they need to complete the trainings.
- Certificates of completion are sent to learners who complete and turn in a "Reflection" worksheet at the end of each

training. The items on the Reflection worksheet address the following areas:

- Brief summary of purpose, objectives, and content
- Request for comments on usefulness of the content in relation to the learner's context and discipline
- Request for specific insights, tools, or strategies from this training that were especially useful
- Request for suggestions on how the training could be enriched or improved

- Over 103 trainings have been completed by local, national, and international learners to date, with new learners signing up each week as the trainings continue to be offered into the future.

- Reflection comments for both courses have been overwhelmingly positive and express appreciation for the opportunity to learn in a flexible, free, and open online environment.

- The vast majority of participants, both inside and outside of nursing, have communicated that the content of these trainings provided new understandings, helpful suggestions and methods, and needed validation about the importance of caring in the digital world in all disciplines and settings.

Pearls of Wisdom

When the infrastructure or support is not available for the creation of a MOOC, or when lower maintenance outreach/teaching methods are preferred, online self-paced trainings provide opportunities for sharing knowledge with broad local, national, and international populations.

REFLECTIONS FROM JEAN WATSON: EXPRESSING GLOBAL INTENT TO CARE THROUGH MOOCs AND OTHER FORMS OF DIGITAL WORLD EDUCATION

The naturalist writer Terry Tempest Williams (2001) reminds us that "the eyes of the future are looking right at us and they are praying for us to see beyond our own time." There are now 7 billion people on this planet, and we in the Cyberworld and the Caritas CyberCaring community have to ask new questions—perhaps sacred questions—about how our presence, our intention, our consciousness, are communicating/radiating Caritas Consciousness beyond time and space and physicality, in harmony with the Universal Field of love. This is our awakening to one world—a universal humanity.

I witness the Caritas Consciousness evolution of nursing all over the world. We all want the same thing, namely, that despite our distances, differences, and backgrounds, which separate us and make the unknown "other" the enemy in our world, CyberCaring unites us individually and collectively. Transcending differences, transcending space and location with a shared consciousness, CyberCaring is allowing for human-to-human and spirit-to-spirit connections and communication not possible previously.

As I engage with global nursing and many of the unique cultures of the world—from the Asian Pacific to the Middle East to Europe, North and South America, to South Africa and beyond—there is *one truth of our shared humanity:* We all want and need love and affection; kindness and support; we all want and need to be "seen"; we all want and need to be heard; we all want to know that what we have to say matters. We also need open space to hear ourselves, express ourselves, and be accepted as unique individuals, deserving of love and dignity—regardless of living condition, history, culture, religion, beliefs, geography, and world or regional/national politics of any given continent.

In the CyberCaring work and world, we aspire to rise above politics and policies, which separate, rather than unite, our hearts and humanity. This becomes a critical sacred CyberCaring position, once we evolve individually and collectively to a higher level of unitary consciousness—this is the new CyberCaring Caritas world.

This CyberCaring Caritas community now has a unique opportunity to serve as a model for the world. Nursing is the largest health profession in the world. Just consider: If we who hold a CyberCaring consciousness and are engaged in CyberCaring become intentional and focused in manifesting lovingkindness and energy into our focused community, we, the CyberCaring community, would be affecting the energetic field of the entire universe.

REFERENCES

Baturay, M. H. (2015). An overview of the world of MOOCs. *Procedia-Social and Behavioral Sciences, 174,* 427–433.

Brahimi, T., & Sarirete, A. (2015). Learning outside the classroom through MOOCs. *Computers in Human Behavior, 51,* 604–609.

Childs, A. (2006). The complex gastrointestinal patient and Jean Watson's Theory of Caring in nutrition support. *Gastroenterology Nursing, 29*(4), 283–288.

Clark, C. (2013). An integral-caring-science RN-BS nursing curriculum: Outcomes from fostering consciousness evolution. *International Journal for Human Caring, 17*(2), 67–76.

Emoto, R., Tsutsui, M., & Kawana, R. (2015). A model to create a caring and healing environment for nurses in child and family nursing. *International Journal for Human Caring, 19*(1), 8–12.

Gustin, L. W., & Wagner, L. (2012). The butterfly effect of caring—clinical nursing teachers' understanding of compassion as a source of compassionate care. *Scandinavian Journal of Caring Sciences,* 27(1), 175–183.

Jones, M., Hendricks, J. M., & Cope, V. (2012). Toward an understanding of caring in the context of telenursing. *International Journal for Human Caring, 16*(1), 7–15.

Meng, M., Xiuwei, Z., & Anli, J. (2011). A theoretical framework of caring in the Chinese context: A grounded theory study. *Journal of Advanced Nursing, 67*(7), 1523–1536.

Ogugu, E., Odero, T, Ong'any, A., & Wagoro, M. (2015). Nurses' and patients' perceptions on the importance of nurse-caring behaviors: A study at the surgical wards of Kenyatta National Hospital, Nairobi. *International Journal for Human Caring, 19*(2), 55–61.

Ozkan, I. A., Okumus, H., Buldukoglu, K., & Watson, J. (2013). A case study based on Watson's Theory of Human Caring: Being an infertile woman in Turkey. *Nursing Science Quarterly, 26*(4), 352–359.

Santos, M. R., Bousso, R. S., Vendramim, P., Baliza, M. F., Misko, M. D., & Silva, L. (2014). The practice of nurses caring for families of pediatric inpatients in light of Jean Watson. *Revista da Escola de Enfermagem da USP, 48*(Esp), 80–86.

Suliman, W. A., Welmann, E., Omer, T., & Thomas, L. (2009). Applying Watson's Nursing Theory to assess patient perceptions of being cared for in a multicultural environment. *Journal of Nursing Research, 17*(4), 293–300.

Watson, J. (1999). *Postmodern nursing and beyond.* London, UK: Churchill Livingstone.

Williams, T. T. (2001). *Red: Passion and patience in the desert.* New York, NY: Pantheon Books.

8

Caring Continuing

In this chapter, you will learn about

- *Maintaining intent to care on a daily basis*
- *Daily caring touchstones*

C aring continuing and growth in Caritas Consciousness requires daily practice. Simply, briefly, and repeatedly returning to your core of caring intent each day will support this process. Religious devotion, centering, breathwork, yoga, prayer, immersion in nature, or other activities that support awareness, inner resolve, and self-care are all helpful. Individuals should choose activities that resonate with personal beliefs and temperament. In this chapter, daily caring touchstones are offered as one way to support this endeavor. These touchstones may be used alone or in conjunction with other activities.

DAILY CARING TOUCHSTONES

Watson (2002) created caring touchstones to help Caritas nurses practice conscious intention for cultivating love and Transpersonal Caring moments throughout the workday. They have been modified here for use in digital world settings. These touchstones are meant to facilitate centering at critical times: right before you begin work, in the middle of the work shift, at the end of the work shift, and at the close of the day. If used daily, these touchstones will help to sustain caring practice. You will find these caring touchstones formatted into a card-sized image for the front side of a card, and the 10 Caritas Processes formatted for the reverse of a card at the end of the Appendix of this book (also in the free online course materials available from springerpub.com/sitzman-mooc). These may be printed (front and back), laminated, and conveniently carried with you for easy reference wherever you happen to be working.

CARING TOUCHSTONES: SETTING INTENTIONALITY AND CONSCIOUSNESS FOR DIGITAL CARING AND HEALING*

CARING IN THE BEGINNING

• Begin the day with silent gratitude; set your intentions to be open to give and receive all that you are here to give and receive this day; intend to bring your full self, in the day-to-day moments of this day; cultivate a loving, caring consciousness toward yourself and all others who enter your path in person and in the digital world.

CARING IN THE MIDDLE

• Take brief quiet moments to "center," to empty out, to be still with yourself before entering into interactions or sending/receiving messages; cultivate a loving–caring consciousness toward each person and each situation you encounter; fully attend to the spirit and humanity of each person who enters your awareness.

• Return to these loving-centered intentions again and again throughout the day, helping yourself to remember why you are here.

• In stressful moments, remember to breathe; ask for guidance when frightened, unsure, confused, or unsettled; forgive and bless each situation.

• Let go of that which you cannot control.

_____
*Adapted from Watson (2002).

CARING IN THE END

- At the end of the day, fold these intentions into your heart; commit yourself to cultivating a loving–caring practice for yourself.

- Use whatever has presented itself to you this day as lessons to teach you to grow more deeply into your own humanity and inner wisdom.

- At the end of the day, offer gratitude for all that has entered the sacred circle of your life and work this day.

- Bless, release, and dedicate the day to a higher, deeper order of the great sacred circle of life.

CARING CONTINUING

- Create your own intentions and your own authentic practices to prepare your Caritas Consciousness and digital caring practices; find your individual spiritual path toward cultivating this in your life and work, and in the world.

Pearls of Wisdom

Pausing for a few moments at the beginning, middle, and end of the day to coax awareness back to your core intent to care will support ongoing inner resolve and illuminate new caring possibilities.

REFLECTIONS FROM JEAN WATSON: DIGITAL CARING CONTINUING

In this last part of the book, I offer a message for your heart; for your hopes and visions you hold for yourself, your caring practices and your engagement in CyberCaring. As we together step into authentic caring in the digital world, we each are seeking new self-caring practices that unite us, that help us learn ways to deepen and sustain this work—personally/professionally/universally.

In CyberCaring, we offer our life and learning—first with self, then one person to another, heart to heart; this is a shared life journey to find more conscious, intentional ways to live Caritas within and without.

HEART WISDOM

You are called to honor the sacred nature of your heart. Your heart is the source for Caring, Compassion, Love, Beauty, Truth—the very source for sustaining your humanity and your humanness.

- Both literally and metaphysically: "*What we carry in our heart matters.*"

- The heart manifests a radiant field 500 times greater than the brain.

- The heart is more than just an organ that pumps blood.

- Heart research acknowledges the heart has its own type of *heart intelligence.*

- The heart sends more messages to the brain than the brain sends to the heart.
- The heart communicates its energetic message nonverbally, energetically into the Universal Field, uniting and connecting us around the globe.

LISTENING TO OUR HEARTS

With this awareness of the heart as source for caring, healing, and love, remember:

"Listening to your heart" is not just a figure of speech. As you connect with your heart and evoke lovingkindness and Caritas from your heart center, you are opening your heart to your inner truth as your inner soul guide.

INVITING CARITAS HEART MEDITATION

The following Caritas heart meditation is an invitation to listen to your heart, knowing your heart is your inner guide. In this meditation, you are evoking, envisioning, and inviting *universal cosmic consciousness of love, compassion, and gratitude as an inner practice.*

To Begin:

Take three very cleansing, relaxing, releasing breaths—

> Release anything in your inner mind and all your thoughts; as you close your mind and your eyes to the outer world, open your eyes to your inner world.

Fully relax your body—fall into your body—let yourself be fully present.

With a quiet mind, say to yourself silently:

"I come to you in the quiet; to be still and to listen to my heart."

In this quiet place, as you continue to breathe, find that still point inside—the space between your breaths—the void empty space between inspiring and expiring.

In this quiet place in your heart center, release any thoughts that come into your mind. Simply breathe gratitude from your heart, appreciating yourself in this quiet space.

Feel how good it is to be still and quiet, opening your heart to a sense of gratitude for your own life and this moment.

Let yourself now fall more deeply, lovingly into your heart— breathing lovingkindness and compassion through your heart.

In this deeper heart space, allow and watch thoughts and feelings rise—any memories, hurts, pains, successes, disappointments, celebrations, sufferings, joys—let your feelings just wash over you without judging, watching your heart opening more and more, letting your heart comfort you. Let the thoughts and feelings rise and fall without following them—just compassionately allowing them to be there.

Returning to loving tender feelings filling up and expanding your heart.

Gently radiate your Caritas heart love feelings to everyone and everything in your life.

Radiate these Caritas heart feelings to others: your family, colleagues, caring community, and your patients.

Hold in your mind's eye images of your heart vibrating ripples of love—visualize violet vibrations rippling into the world— knowing that heart energy of love connects us across distances and time—you are touching the hearts of others, making a silent difference in this moment; in this quiet moment, you are experiencing the Oneness of all.

Radiate Caritas heart love to others—

Far out into the Universal Field of humanity—to anyone and all others in the world who are suffering and in need of caring and love. Envision ripples and waves of the beautiful energy of love—visualize violet—white light vibrations rippling into the world—filling up and surrounding the planet with your heart-centered intentions and silent messages of love—knowing you are not alone. Hearts connect at the nonphysical, spirit level.

Gently and tenderly—energetically—bring these Caritas heart feelings back to yourself.

Wrap these feelings around yourself; let the Caritas heart feelings surround and embrace you.

AND know: **YOU ARE LOVE. WE are ONE!**

Return to your current space; become aware of your surroundings.

Take a deep stretching breath; feel yourself fully embodied, light, and openhearted.

Bow to the universe as a gesture of humility, gratitude, and grace!

Namaste—
May the love and light in my heart
Touch the love and light in your heart
In Caritas, Jean
May you know we are all connected!

REFERENCE

Watson J. (2002). Metaphysics of virtual caring communities. *International Journal for Human Caring.* 6(1), 41–45.

IV

Teaching Materials

9

Course Resources

INSTRUCTOR'S COURSE PLAN

UNIT 1 Dates:	Title: Watson's Caring Science as Context for Digital World Caring Objectives: • Discuss the overall purpose of the text and course. • Describe how mindfulness can be a means of facilitating caring in the digital world. • Define Caritas Consciousness and Transpersonal Caring within the context of the digital world. Readings: Preface, Chapters 1–2 Discussion Question(s): • Please discuss the extent of your current digital world usage (i.e., anything that has to do with sending, receiving, and/or viewing digital world content). • Share one instance in your professional life when digital world caring was evident, and describe how that instance impacted you and the others involved. *Please be sure to maintain privacy for the people involved by *not* posting true names or other detailed identifying information.

UNIT 2 Dates:	Title: Watson's 10 Caritas Processes and How to Apply Them in the Digital World Objectives: • Describe Watson's 10 Caritas Processes • Explain how Watson's 10 Caritas Processes apply to Caring in the digital world Readings: Chapters 3–4 Discussion Question(s): • Share one instance you experienced or were aware of when caring was *not* evident in a digital world situation. • Describe how two or more of the Caritas Processes described in Chapters 3 and 4 could have been employed to support caring in this situation. *Please be sure to maintain privacy for the people involved by *not* posting true names or other detailed identifying information.
UNIT 3 Dates:	Title: Expressing Caring in Digital Classrooms and General Digital Communications • Explain what nurse educators can do to sustain caring in the digital world. • Explain what students can do to sustain caring in the digital world. • Consider how digital caring strategies could be uniquely incorporated into your own teaching/learning activities. • Analyze how the caring digital communication examples in Chapter 6 might be modified to fit within your own communication style and habits. Readings: Chapters 5–6 Discussion Question(s): • Create a list of three digital world social/professional/educational situations that you find challenging. *Please be sure to maintain privacy for people involved by *not* posting true names or other detailed identifying information.

	• For each of the three items on your list, modify/utilize the caring digital communication examples presented in Chapters 5–6 to craft communications/messages that will address each concern within the Transpersonal Caring framework.
UNIT 4 Dates:	Title: Expanding and Continuing Digital World Caring Objectives: Explore how MOOCs and free and open trainings may be used to support the establishment of a collective intent to care on local and global scales. Consider possibilities related to open online content in relation to forging connections across cultures, distance, space, and time on a global scale in nursing and beyond. Create personal strategies for digital caring continuing. Readings: Chapters 7–8 Discussion Question(s): • Perform an Internet search to find examples of nursing-related free and open online courses and MOOCs. Identify topical areas currently not addressed that you would like to see addressed in free and open content (in your organization, community, region, country, and globally) that are not currently available. • Discuss how addressing the topical areas you identified would benefit nurses and others on local and global scales. • Describe personalized strategies for incorporating digital caring into your own daily digital world presence.

SYLLABUS

1. Certificate of Completion issued upon successful completion of the course.

2. Course Type: Online

3. Prerequisites: None. This is an introductory course.

4. Course Description: Learners will be introduced to Watson's Caring Theory and how it can be implemented in the digital world. Exploration and learning related to key concepts will be supported through the introduction of mindfulness practices, reflective narrative, and contemplative art.

5. Course Faculty: Kathleen Sitzman, PhD, RN, CNE, ANEF

6. Course Objectives:

   ■ On completion of this course, the student will be able to:

      i. Describe practical examples that illustrate Watson's 10 Caritas Processes and Transpersonal Caring moments in the digital world.

      ii. Use research-based digital caring practices to convey and sustain caring in online classrooms.

      iii. Apply research-based digital caring communication principles to convey caring in digital world interactions.

      iv. Analyze how free and open digital world content might support collective caring on a global scale.

      v. Discuss how Watson's Caring Touchstones might be useful in everyday professional practice.

7. Teaching Strategies:

   ■ Course-specific reading materials in either print and/or online formats

   ■ Asynchronous online postings and discussion boards

- Online reflective journaling
- Multimedia presentations as appropriate in the online setting

8. Topical Areas:

- Watson's "Human Caring Theory" as context for digital world caring
- Conveying and sustaining caring in digital world learning environments
- Expressing caring in digital communications
- Expressing local and global intent to care through free and open online trainings and courses
- Caring Touchstones for caring continuing

9. Students Are Expected to Demonstrate Academic Integrity:

- Students will do their own work and assist others with course work only when the instructor specifies that group work/collaboration is expected or acceptable.
- Students will not copy the language, structure, and ideas of others and then indicate that they created the work themselves. Students will provide citations when using/discussing the work of others.
- Students will be truthful regarding any circumstances related to academic work.
- Students will treat themselves and others with love, respect, courtesy, and an appreciation for diversity.
- Students will maintain anonymity/privacy related to the situations described in online postings.

10. Evaluation Methods: This class will be pass/fail. Students earning 80% of the total points available in the course will receive a passing grade and earn the corresponding Certificate of Completion.

11. Posting of Grades: All grades will be posted in the course grade book. In compliance with the Family Educational Rights and Privacy Act, grades are not public and will be visible only to individual students and the instructor.

12. Policy on Late Work/Extensions: Extensions of up to 48 hours will generally be allowed for extenuating circumstances on a case-by-case basis.

13. Required Textbook:

    ■ Sitzman, K., Watson, J. (2016). *Watson's Caring in the Digital World: A Guide for Caring When Interacting, Teaching, and Learning in Cyberspace*. New York, NY: Springer Publishing.

COURSE INTRODUCTION

Welcome to class. I look forward to working with you over the next 5 weeks. Here are some suggestions that will help you successfully participate in this course from the beginning through to the end:

1. Explore all of the icons on the course home page because they all have important information that will clarify what you need to do to be successful throughout the duration of the course. Here is a rundown of what each icon offers:

   a. *Syllabus:* This icon takes you to general information about the course.

   b. *Course Calendar:* This icon takes you to the class schedule. Be sure to print it out and carefully note assignment due dates to make sure you keep up with the course.

   c. *Assignment Descriptions:* This icon takes you to the assignment description and rubric information page. Here you will learn what is required to successfully complete each assignment and how you will receive credit for your work.

   d. *Unit Modules:* This icon takes you to weekly organizer buttons. Clicking on one of the weekly organizer buttons will take you to information and helpful links in relation to required units of study for the corresponding week. Within each unit of study, there will be an easy link to corresponding discussion posting and journaling areas.

   e. *Resources:* This icon takes you to links for electronic resources that may be helpful to you.

   f. *Instructor's Office:* This icon takes you to a brief introduction of your instructor that includes important contact information.

   g. *Course Orientation:* You are here right now! I hope it is helping to clarify things!

   h. *Instructor Blog or Announcements:* Click on this icon twice each week, on Mondays and Thursdays, to check for new developments.

2. Print out the course calendar, and fill in the dates that correspond to the weeks listed on the calendar. The date you should fill in for *Week 1* corresponds to the week in which the class begins, and so on.

3. Print out the Instructor information so that you have a hard copy. This way, if the online course page goes down and you have temporarily lost the ability to contact the teacher via the course, you will still have the information you need to contact the teacher in a different way if needed.

4. Familiarize yourself with the units, journaling forums, and posting forums the first day the course opens so that you are able to keep up from the very beginning. Many studies related to online learning have shown that procrastination is one of the most common reasons why students fail online courses.

5. The most successful online students complete a small amount of work on the course each day at a specified time—for instance, during lunch breaks.

6. Do not hesitate to ask for help from me via e-mail or online postings. I want you to be successful, and I am here to help you.

INSTRUCTOR INTRODUCTION

Welcome!

I am Kathleen Sitzman, and I will be your professor for this course. I love teaching in the digital world and look forward to engaging in collaborative teaching/learning with you.

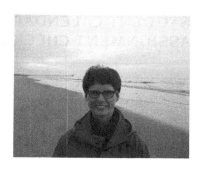

I earned my BSN and MSN degrees from the University of Utah and my PhD from the University of Northern Colorado. My husband and I live near a beach in the southeastern United States. We have been married for 35 years and have three grown children who are all off doing wonderful things. When I am not teaching, I enjoy cooking, sailing, reading, walking, and flying different kinds of kites on the beach.

Please do not hesitate to contact me if you need me. E-mail is the most efficient way to reach me as I check it many times a day during working hours Monday–Friday. My e-mail address is sitzmank@ecu.edu

I enjoy connecting with my students via phone and/or video Skype. If you would like to talk, brainstorm, problem-solve, process, and so forth, then please send an e-mail message to me, indicating a few days/times when you are available, and we will work together to get a phone or video Skype meeting arranged.

I believe we all have something to share that will teach others new and important insights. I am a collaborative partner in this teaching/learning endeavor. I look forward to working with you as we learn together in this course.

Dr. Sitzman

COURSE CALENDAR

STUDENT CALENDAR AND READING/ ASSIGNMENT CHECKLIST

Week 1 Place dates here: _____	**UNIT 1** Title: Watson's Caring Science as Context for Digital World Caring Objectives: • Discuss the overall purpose of the text and course. • Describe how mindfulness can be a means of facilitating caring in the digital world. • Define Caritas Consciousness and Transpersonal Caring within the context of the digital world. Readings: Preface, Chapters 1–2 Complete this assignment checklist: • Please discuss the extent of your current digital world usage (i.e., anything that has to do with sending, receiving, and/or viewing digital world content). • Share one instance in your professional life when digital world caring was evident, and describe how that instance impacted you and the others involved. *Please be sure to maintain privacy for the people involved by *not* posting true names or other detailed identifying information. • Your main posting that addresses the two questions above can be in first-person narrative (250 or more words). • Thoughtfully respond to at least two classmates' online postings.

	Assessment: The assignments that you will post on the Unit 1 discussion board are worth 50 points and will be assessed based on the following rubric:

Required Element	Points Possible
First-person narrative response genuinely and thoughtfully explains connections to unit content, objectives, and readings	**25**
Thoughtful online response to a minimum of two classmates	**10**
Grammar and spelling	**10**
Netiquette observed	**5**

Week 2 Place dates here: _____	**UNIT 2** Title: Watson's 10 Caritas Processes and How to Apply Them in the Digital World Objectives: • Describe Watson's 10 Caritas Processes. • Explain how Watson's 10 Caritas Processes apply to caring in the digital world. Readings: Chapters 3–4 Complete this assignment checklist: • Share one instance you experienced or were aware of when caring was *not* evident in a digital world situation. • Describe how two or more of the Caritas Processes described in Chapters 3–4 could have been employed to support caring in this situation.

- *Please be sure to maintain privacy for the people involved by *not* posting true names or other detailed identifying information.
- Your main posting that addresses the two questions above can be in first-person narrative (250 or more words).
- Thoughtfully respond to at least two classmates' online postings.

Assessment: The assignments that you will post on the Unit 2 discussion board are worth 50 points and will be assessed based on the following rubric:

Required Element	Points Possible
First-person narrative response genuinely and thoughtfully explains connections to unit content, objectives, and readings	**25**
Thoughtful online response to a minimum of two classmates	**10**
Grammar and spelling	**10**

Week 3
Place dates here:

_____

UNIT 3
Title: Expressing Caring in Digital Classrooms and General Digital Communications

- Explain what nurse educators can do to sustain caring in the digital world.
- Explain what students can do to sustain caring in the digital world.
- Consider how digital caring strategies could be uniquely incorporated into your own teaching/learning activities.
- Analyze how the caring digital communication examples in Chapter 6 might be modified to fit within your own communication style and habits.

Readings: Chapters 5–6
Complete this assignment checklist:

- Create a list of three digital world social/professional/ educational situations that you find challenging. *Please be sure to maintain privacy for people involved by *not* posting true names or other detailed identifying information.
- For each of the three items on your list, modify/utilize the caring digital communication examples presented in Chapters 4–5 to craft communications/messages that will address each concern within the Transpersonal Caring framework.
- Your main posting that addresses the two questions above can be in first-person narrative (250 or more words).
- Thoughtfully respond to at least two classmates' online postings.

Assessment: The assignments that you will post on the Unit 3 discussion board are worth 50 points and will be assessed based on the following rubric:

Required Element	Points Possible
First-person narrative response genuinely and thoughtfully explains connections to unit content, objectives, and readings	**25**
Thoughtful online response to a minimum of 2 classmates	**10**

Week 4 Place dates here: _____	**UNIT 4** Title: Expanding and Continuing Digital World Caring Objectives:
	<ul><li>Explore how MOOCs and free and open trainings may be used to support the establishment of a collective intent to care on local and global scales.</li><li>Consider possibilities related to open online content in relation to forging connections across cultures, distance, space, and time on a global scale in nursing and beyond.</li><li>Create personal strategies for digital caring continuing.</li></ul> Readings: Chapters 6–7 Complete this assignment list: <ul><li>Perform an Internet search to find examples of nursing-related free and open online courses and MOOCs. Identify topical areas currently not addressed that you would like to see addressed in free and open content (in your organization, community, region, country, and globally) that are not currently available.</li><li>Discuss how addressing the topical areas you identified would benefit nurses and others on local and global scales.</li><li>Express your personalized strategies for incorporating digital caring into your own daily digital world presence. You have the option to use first-person narrative response, **OR** you have the option to use pointillism, mandala, or photographic images to represent your thoughts and feelings.</li><li>Your main posting that addresses the two questions above can be in first-person narrative (250 or more words).</li><li>Thoughtfully respond to at least two classmates' online postings.</li></ul>

Assessment: The assignments that you will post on the Unit 4 discussion board are worth 50 points and will be assessed based on the following rubric:

Required Element	Points Possible
First-person narrative response genuinely and thoughtfully explains connections to unit content, objectives, and readings **OR** Pointillism, mandala, or photographic image shows effort, creativity, and a genuine, heartfelt connection to required content. The brief explanation should clarify your intent in creating the image.	**25**
Thoughtful online response to a minimum of 2 classmates	**10**
Grammar and spelling	**10**
Netiquette observed	**5**

ASSIGNMENT CLARIFICATION AND GRADING

ASSIGNMENT SUMMARY

Total Points Available in the Course:

Required Discussion Board Postings: 4 @ 50 points each = 200

1. Class will be pass/fail. Students earning 80% of the total points available in the course will receive a passing grade and earn the corresponding Certificate of Completion.

Grading Criteria:
Passing Grade = 160 points and above

Failing Grade = 159.9 points and below

Assignment Clarification:
Discussion Board Postings (200 Points): Regular and committed participation is integral to successful completion of this interactive course. A significant amount of knowledge development will occur through group discussion, sharing, and collaboration. It is essential for you to read the assigned chapters and consider how they apply to your experiences.

Discussion board postings will involve each student providing online responses to unit content, and thoughtfully responding to the postings of others in the class. Substantive, thoughtful, and well-constructed postings are expected. Reading the unit chapters, reading the postings of classmates, forming opinions, and then mindfully communicating your thoughts are all required for success in this endeavor. Empowered student communication forms the basis for all discussions. The underlying philosophy of this approach is to embrace diversity, hear every voice, and respect each group member. In this process, the focus is on valuing what is shared among our teaching/learning colleagues. Courtesy, respect, and restraint are hallmarks of this approach. Please read the Digital Caring Etiquette handout in this course as you will be responsible for demonstrating these behaviors throughout the duration of this course.

Please maintain anonymity/privacy related to the situations described in your postings.

2. Here is an example of the point breakdown: There are 50 points possible for *each* of the 4 learning units—one per week for 4 weeks (200 points total). The 50 points possible per unit are broken down in this way: There are 25 points possible for your scholarly response to each unit question and 10 points possible for your scholarly responses to a minimum of two classmate postings within each unit. Grammar and spelling are worth 10 points, and proper use of netiquette is worth an additional 5 points (total = 50). Further explanation: Let us say you are in Week 1 of this course and have just completed the readings associated with Unit 1 of Week 1. If you go to the discussion board area for Week 1 Unit 1, create and post a substantive response to the Unit 1 content, and then thoughtfully respond to two classmates' postings, using appropriate grammar, spelling, and netiquette, then you will earn 50 points (perfect score) for the required Unit 1 discussion board posting assignment. Let us continue by saying that your twin sister is also in the course and she forgets to spell check, thereby misspelling five words somewhere in her postings (-5 points), and she also responds to only one classmate instead of two (-5 points), so she ends up earning 40 points for the same unit.

Here is a grading rubric for Units 1 to 3 discussion postings:

Required Element	Points Possible
First-person narrative response genuinely and thoughtfully explains connections to unit content, objectives, and readings	**25**
Thoughtful online response to a minimum of two classmates	**10**
Grammar and spelling	**10**
Netiquette observed	**5**

Here is a grading rubric for the Unit 4 discussion posting:

Required Element	Points Possible
First-person narrative response genuinely and thoughtfully explains connections to unit content, objectives, and readings **OR** Pointillism, mandala, or photographic image shows effort, creativity, and a genuine, heartfelt connection to required content. The brief explanation should clarify your intent in creating the image.	**25**
Thoughtful online response to a minimum of two classmates	**10**
Grammar and spelling	**10**
Netiquette observed	**5**

DIGITAL CARING ETIQUETTE GUIDELINES

DIGITAL CARING ETIQUETTE

Please…

1. Spell and grammar check before sending or posting anything.

2. Use a polite greeting at the beginning of messages, such as, "Hello Dr. Sitzman…" or "Dear AnneMarie…"

3. Close messages and postings with your name so that readers can be certain of who wrote it. In professional or academic settings, use your first and last name.

4. Never use all capital letters in any message or posting as this could be perceived as shouting.

5. Use black font that is easy to read.

6. Adopt the practice of writing "please" and "thank you" wherever possible.

7. Never post or text private or sensitive content.

8. Never post or text identifying information or *any* images of clients, patients, colleagues, or work situations.

9. Never use social media to discuss or post images of clients, patients, colleagues, or work situations.

10. Treat every digital experience and activity as an opportunity to care.

CARING TOUCHSTONES

Caring in the Beginning: Begin the day with silent gratitude; set your intentions to be open to give and receive all that you are here to give and receive this day; intend to bring your full self, in each moment of this day; cultivating a loving, caring consciousness toward self and all others who enter your path.

Caring in the Middle: Take brief quiet moments to "center," to empty out, to be still with yourself before entering into interactions or sending/receiving messages; cultivate a loving-caring consciousness toward each situation you encounter; fully attend to the spirit and humanity of each person who enters your awareness.

Return to these loving-centered intentions again and again throughout the day, helping yourself to remember why you are here.

In the middle of stressful moments, remember to breathe; ask for guidance when frightened, unsure, confused, or unsettled; forgive and bless each situation.

Let go of that which you cannot control.

Caring in the End: At the end of the day, fold these intentions into your heart; commit yourself to cultivating a loving-caring practice for yourself.

Use whatever has presented itself this day as lessons to teach you to grow more deeply into your own humanity and inner wisdom.

At the end of the day, offer gratitude for all that has entered the sacred circle of your life and work this day.

Bless, release, and dedicate the day to a higher, deeper order of the great sacred circle of life.

Caring Continuing: Create your own intentions and authentic practices to develop your *Caritas Consciousness;* find your own spiritual path in support of this work. (Copyright Jean Watson 2002)

WATSON'S 10 CARITAS PROCESSES

1. Embrace altruistic values and practice lovingkindness with self and others.

2. Instill faith and hope and honor others.

3. Be sensitive to self and others by nurturing individual beliefs and practices.

4. Develop helping-trusting-caring relationships.

5. Promote and accept positive and negative feelings as you authentically listen to another's story.

6. Use creative scientific problem-solving methods for caring decision making.

7. Share teaching and learning that addresses individual needs and comprehension styles.

8. Create a healing environment for the physical and spiritual self that respects human dignity.

9. Assist with basic physical, emotional, and spiritual human needs.

10. Open to mystery and allow miracles to enter. (Sitzman & Watson, 2014)

Index

Printed in the United States
by Baker & Taylor Publisher Services